The BUTCHER of Rosebank

A real life Dr. Jekyll and Mr. Hyde

a **JON ABBOTT** investigation

Published by Jon Abbott, Kommetjie, South Africa
ISBN: 978-0-620-89984-0 (Paperback)
ISBN: 978-0-620-96191-2 (Ebook)

Published by Perspective Publications

Email: Dearjon@webafrica.org.za

Layout and cover by Boutique Books

Cover: Mariskca du Plessis.
At the age of 14, Mariskca was sentenced to life in a wheelchair by Dr. Lieberthal's butchery.

Dedication

To Gayle—the Best Wife Ever

Acknowledgements

Thanks to Rosemarie Lewis for editing and proofreading

By the same author

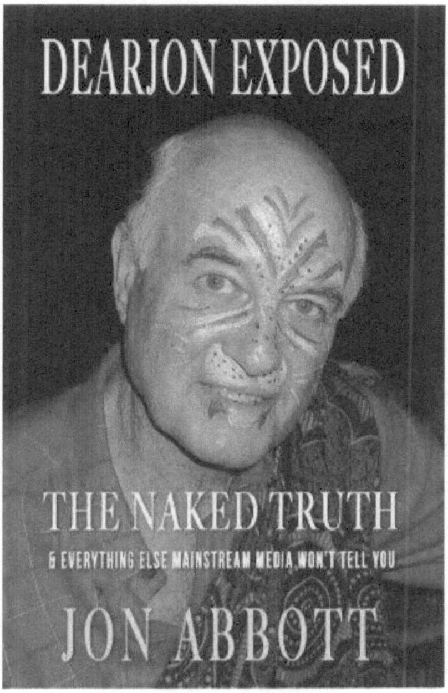

CONTENTS

Chapter 1

Maliza

It was hard to imagine what kind of trauma this 14-year-old girl was going through as she came round. With her mind already in turmoil, her anxiety was heightened to near panic by what she saw when her stepfather helped a nurse turn her.

She asked them to do this because she was so sore on the one side. To her horror, the bed was a sea of blood beneath her.

Despite her young age, having a back operation was nothing new to her, but she had never felt as scared as this before. In tears, she kept imploring her stepfather to promise that she would not be paralyzed.

She had just had what she was told would be a routine operation by spinal specialist Dr. Wynne Lieberthal. He was so highly thought of at the Johannesburg Hospital that she had no reason to think that it would be any different to the others she had there. Everything changed soon afterwards. While her parents were desperately trying to contact him, they were shocked by what they read in a newspaper.

Years earlier, another young girl had to face the same frightening prospect. She too woke desperately worried whether she would ever walk again after Lieberthal had operated on her, unaware that he was still a trainee orthopedic surgeon.

He was making a name for himself as the shining star of the Wits Medical School's 1992 orthopedic class. Einhard Erken, the Professor Emeritus who headed the Department of Orthopedic Surgery there and at the Johannesburg Hospital, described him as "one of the most brilliant registrars the Department ever trained."

Lieberthal had obtained his initial medical degree at the University of the Witwatersrand in 1979; ran his own GP practice and then he set his sights on becoming what he had always dreamt of, a top spinal surgeon; somebody who had the skill to relieve the tremendous mental and physical agony experienced by back sufferers.

He had an affinity for this kind of pain because he had undergone three back operations himself by the time he became a fully-fledged surgeon. It had exacerbated his anguish because his second operation was what he himself described as a "dismal failure".

"The pain was so unbearable and unrelenting that I agreed to undergo further revision surgery," was what he told colleagues.

Unlike many surgeons, he knew from a patient's point of view just what they went through and what could go wrong. He would surely have the utmost sympathy for anybody in a similar position. With his lofty academic achievements, what more could anybody want in a surgeon.

Sister Denise Vos, who later worked with him in the theatre at the privately owned Rosebank Clinic, also had a lot of good things to say about him. That was when he had his own orthopedic practice.

"He was so good in many ways," she said. "He never fumbled and messed around like some surgeons do. He really worked beautifully."

She talked of an occasion when the gardener at the townhouse complex where she lived had been badly injured in a taxi accident. A pin was put in his leg at the state-run Johannesburg General Hospital, but the leg was still not right. "So I said to Wynne, 'He's a good gardener, and it's such a lengthy business to get these people sorted out at the Gen. Can you do anything for him." Without hesitation he replied, 'I tell you what: bring him to my rooms." He examined him and sent him for x-rays at his expense. He was so good to him, you know."

He stood out in the theatre as the perfect gentleman, she said. Whereas there were other surgeons whose boorish juvenile behavior, including swearing at the nurses and throwing bloody swabs at them. There were evidently more reasons than one for putting patients under in this environment.

"The staff liked working with him in the theatre," she continued. "They were very loyal to him and every year he would give the people who were involved with him in theatre and the girls in his ward a wonderful Christmas party at his home. If he went to Australia, he would bring his staff T-shirts and things like that. He was nice.

"He was so good in many ways. I'm a great reader, but I couldn't afford to buy the latest books all the time. So he always came with a paper bag for me. He would say, 'Look, I've just finished with these books, they are the latest." And I would return them after I had read them."

Lieberthal's finest academic year was 1996 when he graduated as an orthopedic surgeon and became a Fellow of the College of Surgeons of South Africa. He had won award after award while in training.

Academically, there was not much more that he could have achieved.

In between being lauded by his profession, Lieberthal was busy in operating theatres perfecting his skills. It was while doing one of his rounds in the Johannesburg Hospital that he came across twelve-year-old Maliza Booysen.

She had a history of unexplained headaches in 1993 when she and her parents Leonie and Kobus Booysen moved from Kuruman in the north of the Cape Province to Alberton, on the outskirts of Johannesburg, where Maliza became a pupil at President Steyn Primary school.

"When I was in Standard 3, I weighed 23 kilograms," Maliza recalled. "That's how ill I was." Her parents were being driven to distraction by the inability of medical science to put a name to their daughter's mystery illness.

A helpful mother of one of Maliza's school friends suggested she see Dr. Johan Pretorius, a local pediatrician. Lack of money was a problem because the business Kobus started didn't work out and Mrs. Booysen had been forced to leave the accounting job she had only recently got to look after Maliza.

When Leonie took her daughter for the appointment, she was embarrassed to have to say that she did not have the money to pay Pretorius. "Don't worry about the money," said the kindly specialist, who agreed to waive his fee. When he saw Maliza he said to Leonie in Afrikaans, "*God vrou, hou lank is hierdie kind so?*" (God woman, how long has this child been like this?).

After examining Maliza, Pretorius sent her for an MRI scan at his expense. At that time, MRI"s cost around R2 000. At last it seemed they were going to be told what was wrong with their sickly daughter. "We think she's got tuberculosis of the spine," was the doctor's verdict. "And as you haven't got a medical aid, I'm going to refer her to the Johannesburg Hospital for her to see Professor Erken, but she must be admitted immediately."

The following day, Maliza went into the hospital. Five blood tests were done, both at this provincial hospital and at a private one. In every case, the diagnosis was tuberculosis.

She pointed out to me that, as the Johannesburg Gen was a teaching hospital, different doctors saw her all the time. "I was given 13 pills a day for this tuberculosis of my spine," added this slightly built, dark-haired girl who was now aged 25.

Once she left the hospital, she had to go for check-ups every three months. This went on for nine months. In the meantime, her mother managed to get a part-time job at Absa Bank. One day, Leonie's sister-in-law phoned her at work to tell her Maliza had taken a turn for the worse.

"I thought, bugger this I'm going to take Maliza back to Johannesburg General and I want to see Dr. Erken," her mother decided. "He must tell me what's going on, not the ward doctors. When we arrived there, Dr. Erken's secretary told us he wasn't available, but a ward doctor would see Maliza. 'I don't want a ward doctor,' I told her. 'I'm sick and tired of this. I want Dr. Erken.'" Despite her protests, a ward doctor did see her.

Maliza joined in with, "I just want to tell you I was paralyzed at that time. I had no movement from the waist down. I had been like that for three months." Her dad attached wheels to one of their plastic garden chairs to enable her to get around.

The ward doctor put her into bed and minutes later he was called to the phone. He returned to the ward, followed by another doctor. "Wynne, I'm so glad you're here," he said. "I want you to have a look at this child."

Leonie and Maliza were impressed by the sympathetic approach of this new doctor. The thorough way he questioned Maliza gave them hope that, at long last, a cure would be found for her debilitating illness. "Mrs. Booysen, do the blood tests really show that it's tuberculosis?" he asked.

"Yes," she replied.

They were surprised to hear him say, "I don't know what it is, but it's not tuberculosis."

By just questioning the girl, Lieberthal had ruled out what five blood tests had shown. He decided another MRI scan was needed. And when Leonie again couldn't pay, he said, "Don't worry. I'm going to send you to Linksfield Clinic. I want you to take that child there immediately. If I'm busy doing an operation, you wait for me because I want to see that scan. Whatever you do, don't let Maliza stand. She must lie down at all times."

At Linksfield, a privately owned hospital, they were waiting outside the theatre when Lieberthal and another doctor emerged looking at the new scan. Would they get the correct diagnosis this time, they must have wondered? She hadn't got TB. That had been a surprise after all the positive tests.

What Lieberthal said next must have far outweighed their initial relief.

"Mrs. Booysen, Maliza has a tumor, a slow-growing tumor that is eating the spine just below her neck." It was far worse than they could possibly have imagined, especially as Maliza was still so young.

Lieberthal wanted to admit her to the Johannesburg General immediately, but as he still had to book a bed and see when a theatre would be available, he told her mother to take her home until he could make the necessary arrangements. He implored Leonie to make sure her daughter was very well looked after because there was a danger of her being permanently paralyzed. "I've got to go to a conference in Durban, but I'll organize everything. I'll keep in touch."

That was on a Friday and he phoned Leonie that evening to tell her he could not get a theatre until the following Monday. "She's been sick for so long these few days won't harm her," he said. "But please look after her carefully."

The mother and daughter might have been fearful of what the future held, but their spirits were lifted by the exceptional interest this new doctor was showing in Maliza's welfare.

He said he was going to try and get a doctor from Cape Town and another one from Durban to assist him. "I don't know if he did," said Leonie, who must have turned a lot of heads in her younger days. "I didn't care, just as long as my daughter was in good hands. He was the first doctor who was really going to do something for her."

On the Monday, while Maliza was being prepared for theatre, Lieberthal warned her mother that any operation could be dangerous, but he was going to do his best. In an eight-hour procedure, part of one of Maliza ribs was used to build up her spine at the place where the tumor was removed.

When Maliza came out of the theatre, Lieberthal arranged for her mother to sleep in the hospital that night. They were referring to each other now as "Leonie" and "Doctor." They moved her daughter into the Intensive Care Unit to recover and then into a ward. Nobody yet knew whether Lieberthal's efforts had been a success. He felt that divine intervention was needed.

Leonie was instructed to go into her daughter's room; get on her knees and pray. "We can only find out if this child can walk when she wakes up," Lieberthal told her.

It was quite a while before he came into the ward and sat on Maliza's bed. She was very sore. A morphine drip in her arm enabled her to control the dose herself, depending on her pain level.

"This is the test, Maliza," she heard him say. "If you can move your toes, you'll be able to walk again."

All three of them looked at them anxiously. Maliza and her mother's greatest fear was that she would be permanently disabled from the waist down. Then, almost imperceptibly, they began to show signs of life.

"Thank God it's a success," the doctor exclaimed. He was the first to drop his emotional guard. He burst into tears, which set the two women off as well.

"That doctor cared so much," said Maliza. "He was working through that whole experience with me. He was at my side the whole time. He held my hands when I took my first step. He helped me out of bed and put this tube by my side. It was the first time I had been able to walk in three months because no other doctors at the Johannesburg General had been willing to help me."

Where had Professor Erken been? I couldn't understand how this trainee surgeon had been allowed to do such a major spinal operation without any qualified orthopedic specialist having first verified Lieberthal's diagnosis and then been present during the operation.

The answer to this question would explain whether or not Lieberthal had kept to his employment conditions that had been laid down by the Medical Council.

From what Leonie said, it seemed that Lieberthal had diagnosed the tumor without any help and had also made the decision to operate. She obviously didn't know who had assisted him in the theatre, but she never mentioned that any other doctor had spoken to her or seen her daughter.

What happened to the growth? It wasn't malignant thankfully, and Lieberthal handed it over in a bottle.

Their euphoria did not last long. About three weeks after the operation, when Maliza went for a checkup, Lieberthal ordered more x-rays before deciding to do another operation using bone from the bone bank this time. This was another failure, so six months after that he operated again.

He was full of apologies. "Leonie, I'm sorry it didn't work," he told her. "There's nothing else we can do other than put screws in."

Her body had apparently rejected the bone. By the time it came to the third operation, the family had a medical aid so her mother refused to let her go back to the Johannesburg Hospital. It was terrible, she claimed. She slept on the floor to be there to comfort her daughter. It was "dirty, with cockroaches all over the place."

On the third occasion, a metal cage was inserted to keep Maliza's spine together.

She still had a pronounced curvature of the spine that developed because she started walking with her hands on her knees when her legs showed signs of becoming paralyzed. "From that, I still get the odd spasm," she told me. "It's something I live with. My back scar is very, very neat. There's one where my rib was taken out and an even bigger one where they put a pipe in my lung. I used to be very self-conscious about these. Well, of course a girl would be, but not anymore. If it wasn't for Dr. Lieberthal, I wouldn't be here today. He saved my life."

Her recovery was such that in 2007 she was a Latin American ballroom instructor. She danced competitively, and so did her students. She was studying a marketing course at Johannesburg University while working at a training company.

Should Lieberthal, as a learner surgeon, have performed these extensive operations on Maliza with no supervision? "I doubt that he would do an extraordinary, big operation like that on his own unless he projected himself to the family as the surgeon," Professor Jerry George told me, laughing. George became the Professor in charge of the Orthopedic Department after Erken retired in 2002.

He was a Senior Consultant specializing in orthopedics for children when Lieberthal was training. He would have students like Lieberthal under his supervision for four-month stints, and then they would move on. Originally from Poland, he spoke English in a charming, picturesque fashion.

At about the time of Maliza's operation, he told me, orthopedic surgeon James Craig, a "very well-known figure," was treating children part-time at the Johannesburg Hospital where he also taught the registrars.

"He was very strict. He would do the whole operation himself. He would examine the patient before. He would come to visit afterwards, but then follow-up later on would be carried on by a registrar. That's a possibility."

What the Booysens did not know was that Lieberthal was no ordinary registrar when he operated on Maliza. He had a spooky skeleton in his cupboard, which was certainly not for student demonstration purposes. It had resulted in him being ordered to have extra special supervision under Professor Erken's wing.

In 2008, I tried to find out from Professor Erken what the correct procedure should have been with Maliza. He was decidedly uncooperative. "I have no interest anymore. Is it in connection with Wynne Lieberthal?"

'Yes, it is,' I replied.

"No, I'm not really getting into that."

The medical big wigs, who had showered Lieberthal with prizes, might have been less impressed had they known about the shameful life of his Mr. Hyde side that had been going on furtively right under their noses.

This was early in the surgeon's career that was to be so pockmarked with horrifying controversy; well before that other young girl found herself going into theatre, oblivious to his true background.

Chapter 2

Sensational Photograph

In 1955, Vryburg was a dusty little town, or *dorp* as the Afrikaners called them, in the Cape Province. Steeped in Afrikanerdom, it had a concentration camp cemetery for the Boers who died in the Anglo Boer War with a memorial that was erected in 1929. It seemed an unlikely place to find an English speaking Jewish family, especially as a lot of Afrikaners had been pro Hitler during World War II. But Vryburg had a Jewish population of about forty-five families when Wynne Lieberthal and his twin brother Hugh were born there.

Their mother Anita, or Nita, as she was known to friends and family, was then 35 with two other sons, Mervyn aged ten and Isidore who was seven. They lived in the center of the town while Samuel, the 43-year-old head of the family, ran the Double Crown Yeast factory, which also made soap. This was the family business founded by his father Simon, who arrived there in 1911.

In 1960, the five-year-olds began their schooling at Vryburg Primary School. One of their teachers, Marie Sussman, was a farmer's widow living in Cape Town when I spoke to her.

"I taught them in Standard four," she said. "Wynne was a very bright boy. It's such a pity the way things turned out. He was far brighter than Hugh. That's why their Mom told me she was so happy that they were separated when they went into high school because Hugh was able to come into his own then. He had always been overshadowed by his brother."

Wynne and Hugh went up together to the Vryburg Hoerskool.

Toward the end of the sixties, the Lieberthals relocated 200 kilometers away to the bigger town of Klerksdorp. The town was surrounded by gold mines with such famous names as Vaal Reefs, Stilfontein and Buffelsfontein, and the yellow dumps that went with them. The family soap factory had closed, and they moved because they had "financial problems."

In Klerksdorp, Nita worked in a crockery bazaar.

"She was the driving force in the family," Sussman explained. "I heard that Sam was running a mine concession store. I last saw Nita in about 1997, six months before she died of cancer. They were living in Johannesburg then. Sam had died a bit before that. He had been working for Hugh."

At the 900-pupil Milner High School in Klerksdorp, the only English medium school in the area, Lieberthal did well. He was particularly good at sport and in his final year he was in the cricket and rugby first teams. He was also a member of the school's camera club.

It was his interest in photography that led to the first of many newspaper headlines long after he had left school. It was the kind of publicity that would make most people cringe.

The brainy boy got a first class passed in his matriculation examination.

Some years later when industrial psychologist Barbara Donaldson was asked to assess him for the purposes of an insurance claim he was making, he inflated his results considerably. She was misled still further by being told he was elected "vice-head boy" at Milner", despite the fact that he had only entered the school the year before.

In truth, he was enrolled at the school in 1969. The school magazine for 1972, which was his final year, listed him as a prefect. Ronald Bartie was head of the boy's side of this co-ed school and his deputy was Deon Pistorius.

Bartie subsequently became headmaster of the General Smuts High School in Vereeniging in 1995, and it was there twelve years later that I asked him about Lieberthal.

"He was an extrovert type and I have good memories of him. He went to Wits University, I think, while I was at another university, so we didn't meet or have any contact after that. I know he was involved in medical things and so on.

"I saw it in the papers, unfortunately," he added ominously.

The year after he obtained his medical degree, Lieberthal joined the South African Defence Force to do his two year compulsory National Service. He told Donaldson that he served for a year and achieved lieutenant status. His second year was deferred to enable him to specialize in surgery.

Like he did with his matric results, Lieberthal embellished his time in the army in his conversation with Donaldson. Her reports were often sought by the legal fraternity in civil claims where an expert's opinion on the employability of the claimant was required.

She revealed that Lieberthal told her that when doctor volunteers were needed for border duty, he volunteered. Together with 52 other doctors he underwent a stringent selection process involving physical and emotional stress tests. He was one of two doctors selected for 32 Battalion and saw active service in Angola.

32 "Buffalo" Battalion was South Africa's most elite fighting unit. According to the Battalion Veterans Association's website, it was known as "The Terrible Ones" because of its operational successes from its inception in 1975 until it was disbanded in 1993, the year before a democratically elected

government came to power in South Africa. It was the most feared unit in the South West African and Angolan war which took place against the backdrop of the Cold War.

Shrouded in secrecy, the battalion was employed in Angola as a buffer between the regular forces of the South African Defence Force and its Communists enemies. It played an important part in assisting Jonas Savimbi's guerrilla movement UNITA against the Cuban backed forces. Veterans claimed 32 Battalion became legendary among friend and foe and was the most decorated SADF unit since World War II.

The website contains this warning headed: *Dishonesty & Shame*. "There are hordes of people out there who have knowingly discredited our unit without fact or have falsely claimed to have served with 32 Battalion. Some have wicked stories that would frighten even the most hardened of vets. Among these "wannabes" are individuals that share the common denominator of dishonesty and spice up their true role while serving with or sometimes even just in the vicinity of 32 Battalion in a supportive or other capacity.

"During the course of the Battalion's existence there were many people who passed through the unit, but only a few of these individuals actually participated in operations with 32 Battalion, and even less saw any action. This message is intended to caution those individuals who by deed, word or media tarnish the name of 32 Battalion and dishonor all those members who bravely served in the Battalion."

Jay Nel, the Veterans Association's secretary, was unable to find any evidence that Lieberthal had ever been in 32 Battalion. "I have been in contact with a number of people and I think we can say the guy's an imposter.

"2Lt/Dr. Wynne Lieberthal was declared medically unfit in 1984 while stationed at SAMS HQ. That is what we have found to date," said Nel, who was a non-commissioned officer in the unit until 1981. SAMS was the Medical Service, which had its headquarters in Pretoria, South Africa's administrative capital, a very long way from the fighting in Angola.

My urologist, Paul Porteous, told me he heard Lieberthal had claimed that, while serving in Angola, his unit got lost. They hijacked a vehicle which crashed badly, injuring a high ranking South West African People's Organisation (SWAPO) officer traveling inside it.

There and then, in the bush, Lieberthal operated on the man and removed his spleen, thus saving his life. They were subsequently airlifted out by helicopter and, under interrogation, the officer revealed valuable information that enabled the SADF to destroy bases in Angola.

When he later saw Lieberthal, Porteous asked him if this story was true and while Lieberthal played it down, he did not deny it. In the urologist's opinion, this operation that Lieberthal claimed to have done was hard enough to do in a fully equipped theatre, let alone out in the bush.

Confusion as to what Lieberthal was actually doing in the early eighties was certainly not cleared up by Donaldson's report. It made out that, in 1983,

Lieberthal was training to become a surgeon at the Johannesburg Hospital. In that year, he injured his back in a motor accident and had to have a spinal fusion. This could have been why he was invalided out of the army.

He made a third party insurance claim and was paid R400 000. Grounds for his claim were that, because of the injury, he could no longer continue learning to become a surgeon.

This must have made Lieberthal realize that insurance companies were a gullible lot that could easily be had, especially if you were a doctor. With such a respectable title, who would doubt your honesty?

"In 1985, his back problems had not settled sufficiently for him to cope with the requirements of specialization, so he left to start his own general practitioners practice, despite the fact that this had never been his first choice," Donaldson recorded.

Lieberthal's GP practice was in Lyndhurst, a predominantly Jewish part of Johannesburg. His initial partner, Graham Willies, committed suicide. It was then that he was joined by Doctors Rodney Feinberg and Lawrence Bloomberg.

In his late forties, Feinberg, a dapper little man who recalled events that took place years ago as if they were yesterday, was running the practice on his own in 2007 when I spoke to him. Bloomberg had packed for Perth ten years earlier.

Feinberg never met Willies, but he understood he was gay and he had a boyfriend. "The two of them gassed themselves in their flat in 1988. That's when I was approached to join the practice." By that time, Bloomberg had already become a partner.

Feinberg joined on 8 August 1988. This was a date he "always remembered" because two months later he knew he was in trouble from a financial respect.

"It was just unbelievable what was going on there," he said. "Lieberthal had an accountant, and I went to him and said: these are the issues, here are the facts on paper. The accountant at the time was on Lieberthal's side, so whatever I brought up was labeled fictitious."

Feinberg's allegations remained on hold for a year. It was the sensational photograph that set the flames of discontent alight once again. Lieberthal had carried on his interest in photography from his school days. He was a member of the Jabula Camera Club in Lyndhurst and a respected Fellow of the Photographic Society of Southern Africa.

That was until he entered the Society's National Wild Life Salon's competition.

He used to go on photographic expeditions up to the Kalahari Desert with his dentist buddy Leor Yudelowitz, brother of anesthetist Dr. Avie Yudelowitz.

"They were very close friends, and they spent many, many hours together on these trips to the bush to take photographs," Dr. Feinberg continued. "But the whole friendship fell apart over that photograph."

In 1989, Lieberthal's partners were shocked to see he had made the front page of The Saturday Star in the lead story. It was the kind of report nobody would like to read about somebody they knew. It must have been even more galling to young doctors in a new practice, trying to build a name for themselves in the community as highly respected professionals. The cream of photographers in the Photographic Society was outraged.

The paper boldly proclaimed: *Wild Life Winner* above a smaller headline, saying, "Animals in prize photo are stuffed, say judges."

It disclosed that the photograph Feinberg had talked to me about showed a cobra and a mongoose in mortal combat. The three judges gave Lieberthal's slide the highest marks, and he was awarded the Photographic Salon's first prize that included a floating trophy and a gold medal.

Days later, the judges became suspicious because the sand around the subjects was unruffled as if there had been no scuffle. Specialists from various snake parks, as well as the Natal University biology department and a Transvaal taxidermist, were asked to view the slide.

They were unanimous: the animals were stuffed—and so was the naturalist doctor, well and truly. Even his engaging, persuasive personality would not get him out of this one. Didn't the members of the Medical Council read the papers or were they only concerned with the behavior of doctors in relation to patients, not their general morality?

Lieberthal was disqualified. He resigned from the Society and handed back all the medals he had won in the past. He refused to allow the paper to reproduce the picture because he claimed the publication rights had been sold in the United States. So who else got taken for a ride?

The exhibition was hosted by the Port Elizabeth Camera Club. When he was confronted about it being a fraud, he said, "Yes. Here's my medal back, and goodbye."

Feinberg felt Lieberthal had no reason to cheat. He used to give presentations and his genuine photographic work was good. "For me, that summed up the mental state of the man," he said. "From what I understood, the photograph belonged to Leor. He took it at an exhibition of stuffed animals."

That ended Lieberthal's friendship with Yudelowitz, who left the country not long afterwards to live in London.

After this embarrassing photographic scandal, there was a very tense atmosphere between Feinberg and Lieberthal. "He knew that I knew what his bona fides were," Feinberg went on. "He was a brilliant doctor. He had a big following of patients to the point he could con a patient and tell them anything."

He described Lieberthal as "a real people" person. "Where you have trust, you have confidence, and the next thing, there is a problem. It's a great tragedy that a bright, capable man is like this."

When the practice finally unraveled and Lieberthal walked out, Bloomberg phoned attorney Brian Lebos, whose son Martin had been at medical school with him. Lebos' advice was that he believed they had a fighter on their hands.

The remaining partners were left to sort out complaints from patients over accounts they claimed to have paid. "They would produce the proof which showed they had paid by check but it had not gone into the account of the practice," Feinberg said, warming to the story. "So, we built up a whole case against Wynne. To cut a long story short, he committed fraud by double leasing office equipment and motor vehicles that he leased and sold."

Armed with the correct financial information from the new auditors, Feinberg and Bloomberg had an evening meeting with Lieberthal. He arrived with Advocate Mannie Witz and an attorney, who was Witz's brother-in-law. Lebos was there representing his new clients.

Lieberthal bargained till late that night in an effort to get paid a third of the value of the practice, but the other two refused to budge. "At the end of the day, he was told to just walk away and have no claim against us," said Feinberg. "I was actually quite angry because of the fraud he had committed and things like that. But Brian Lebos said to us, 'One Jewish boy doesn't put another Jewish boy in jail. Leave it to him; he will dig his own grave one day.' And that came from a Lebanese attorney."

The ousted medic left the practice in a "big rush" in November 1989. Almost immediately he cashed in on his friendship with Jeff Hurwitz. He and his father Barney owned the Clinic Holdings hospital group that eventually sold out to Netcare.

They gave him a job as the manager of the Rosebank Clinic working under Jeff, and he started there on 1 January 1990 at a salary of R11 250 a month. According to his contract, Lieberthal was to "manage the hospital taking into account all spheres of operation."

It was strange, to say the least, that he should have been given the position of managing an entire hospital when he had done such a bad job of managing himself. His likeable personality that hid some horrific flaws had done it again.

Chapter 3

Bad Addiction

In 1991, Lieberthal was once again after another insurance windfall. He sued Santam Insurance as the agent for the Government's Multilateral Motor Vehicle Accident Fund for just under R1.3-million. In his particulars of claim, he maintained he injured his back again in 1990 when a car collided with his stationary vehicle. He had to have another back operation involving a fusion of vertebrae and was off work for 48 days.

He claimed damages for "pain and suffering, loss of amenities of life and disablement." It was anticipated that he would have "intermittent lower back pain and discomfort for many years."

It was in relation to this case that Donaldson prepared her medico-legal report.

Lieberthal's deviousness was emphasized still further by Advocate Frank Bashall. Acting for Santam, he compiled notes on what Dr. Feinberg told him in an interview: "Lieberthal was awarded damages in 1983 because he could not become an orthopedic surgeon. Despite this, he did jog and attend gym. Now he is claiming for loss of income because he intends to become an orthopedic surgeon."

Other points made in the notes were that Lieberthal led a very lavish lifestyle.

There were fraudulent double leases that probably helped finance this. Book debts of R159 000 were ceded to Investec Bank, but no money was reflected as having been received for these in the practice.

Feinberg got a copy of the cession and showed it to Lieberthal who denied it contained his signature. Cars and other personal assets were put through the books of the practice.

Lieberthal was using Stopayne and Lexotan, although very little Pethidine was prescribed in the practice, despite a lot being ordered.

Barbara Donaldson wrote that Lieberthal appeared to have been a physically active person before the accident. He enjoyed most sports and was especially keen on marathon running. He now had to give up all activities of a sporting nature. His hobbies were philately, photography, and reading. "But since the accident he only reads occasionally because he has difficulty with prolonged sitting or standing."

Laying on the agony, evidently to increase his chances of a big payout, he told her that operating as a trainee surgeon put so much strain on his back that he was only able to work a 20-hour week. He was not optimistic about being able to work a full day. The first operation he had after the 1990 accident was not a success and he was not keen to have another one. "He is also 'terrified to have it done without analgesics', since this would be necessary in view of his history of addiction. And his financial pressures are such that he cannot afford to take the time off for surgery and subsequent recuperation."

She interviewed him in March 1992 and, in a report a month later, Dr. Sylvain de Miranda wrote, "At the time of the motor accident, which is the subject of the present compensation claim, it is accepted that Dr. Lieberthal had already developed a serious drug dependency."

Dr. de Miranda was the Director and Head of Clinical Services at Phoenix House drug rehabilitation center in Johannesburg. When he saw Lieberthal, he was taking 20 Stopayne tablets a day and 24 milligrams of Lexotan at night. He was also injecting himself with 800 milligrams of Pethidine daily.

According to De Miranda, the very rapid growth of Lieberthal's "very successful" private practice from 1985 to 1989 caused him considerable stress with the result that he took Stopayne tablets for tension headaches. "These tablets are highly dependence-producing," De Miranda maintained.

Lieberthal's use of Stopayne escalated rapidly, and he began taking Lexotan, a Benzodiazepine tranquilizer, in addition. He became addicted to these substances "without consciously recognizing this process." When his partner committed suicide, this led to a further escalation of his "self-medication and addictive process."

Early in 1991, it was decided to admit Lieberthal immediately as an in-patient to Riverfield Lodge, another Johannesburg rehabilitation center, in order for him to receive urgent treatment for his drug abuse. The clinic team soon concluded that he "continues to deny" the extent to which his drug problem was "impairing his functioning."

He refused to follow the center's recommendations that he needed intensive long-term treatment for both his dependency and underlying psychological problems. Were those psychological problems the root cause of the inexplicable events that occurred later in his career? I wondered. After four weeks, the clinic had no choice but to discharge him because he believed that "nothing is wrong."

Despite being advised to give up his medical practice and rather consider a period of prolonged treatment, he was "unable to refrain from his drug abuse." This necessitated his admission to Phoenix House, this time to receive long-term in-patient treatment.

"This admission was effected with the knowledge of the South African Medical and Dental Council (This later became the Health Professions Council of South Africa, but I will refer to it in most cases as the Medical Council)," De Miranda wrote.

On the bright side, De Miranda revealed that Lieberthal responded well to the Phoenix House program. He was most co-operative and participated in all levels of therapy. In view of his progress, they discharged him in August 1991 under strict conditions as laid down in a sworn affidavit.

The restrictions were subsequently confirmed by the President of the Medical Council. "It is my experience that such restrictions usually remain in force for a period of 4 to 5 years, depending on the subject's progress," De Miranda disclosed. "However, even after the lifting of these restrictions it will not be recommended by myself, as the supervising and treating doctor, that Dr. Lieberthal should return to general private practice at any time in the future."

If only that had actually happened.

In the sworn affidavit that De Miranda referred to, Lieberthal undertook to be a good boy in future. He was employed as a full-time surgical assistant at Milpark Hospital and Rosebank Clinic. "I hereby undertake to refrain totally from any self-medication for whatever purpose," he promised. He agreed to attend Phoenix House as an out-patient for regular treatment.

Early in 1992, the President of the Medical Council, dentist Professor Len Becker, decided that Lieberthal could only practice under three conditions. He had to continue as a full-time surgical assistant to surgeons Leonard Nainkin, S.L. Weinstein, and D. Snyders, and carry on being treated by Dr. de Miranda, who had to submit reports on his progress every three months. He was prohibited from prescribing drugs in Schedules 5, 6 and 7, which were the highest categories available.

Just eight months later, Professor Erken wrote to Nico Prinsloo, the Registrar of the Medical Council, saying that he had accepted Lieberthal as an orthopedic registrar at the Wits Medical School. "I have spoken to Dr. de Miranda and he agrees that it will be good for him to be a trainee in an academic department."

Had Wits or the Medical Council done a credit check on the doctor Erken was keen to employ, it would have found that the skeleton in Lieberthal's cupboard had a lot more diseased bones than just a drug problem.

Lieberthal sent a letter to Prinsloo saying he had made excellent progress in the last 16 months and he had not, in any way, transgressed his restrictions. He had registered to write the first part of his Surgical Fellowship exam through the College of Medicine of South Africa.

During his time as a surgical assistant, he had been exposed to all types of narcotic analgesics, sedatives, and tranquillizers, which were freely available in any theatre. Furthermore, pharmaceutical reps regularly called on the theatre complex, handing out samples of all types of drugs but, since his initial therapy, he had "not once relapsed" and he certainly had "no intention nor desire to do so."

He was due to start a registrar's post in Prof Erken's department of Orthopedic Surgery on 1 September 1992. This post would be at the Hillbrow Hospital. It carried "a certain amount of seniority and an enormous amount of responsibility".

The position would require him to give urgent treatment for such things as fractured bones and post-operative pain. To do this, he would need to administer scheduled analgesics and sedatives. Due to the structure of the academic circuit, he would, at all times, be ultimately responsible to a senior consultant, but would have to do initial assessments and treatment himself.

"I will therefore need your permission to prescribe analgesics such as Pethidine, Omnopon, and oral analgesic preparations like Propain Forte, as well as sedatives and hypnotics such as Valium and Serepax," he stated.

To enable him to prescribe these drugs in his new job, he asked that his restrictions on prescribing Schedule 5, 6 and 7 drugs be lifted as soon as possible. He gave the following undertakings: "I am even prepared to prescribe them only within the hospital environment. I am also fully prepared to have this reviewed as frequently as you deem necessary and am willing to subject myself to regular random urine testing, daily if necessary."

Despite his Santam insurance claim not yet being finalized, his letter stated, "I am enjoying excellent physical and mental health and my personal and family relationships are excellent."

This did not tally with what he told psychiatrist Dr. David Shevel when he had a second consultation with him in January 1993 in connection with his 1990 injury that was the basis of his second accident claim. This was only four months after he wrote his letter to Prinsloo.

"Dr. Lieberthal informs me that he still has pain in his lower back and a tingling sensation in his left leg and foot," Shevel reported. "He uses Panado and Brufin if the backache is very severe. Emotionally, he is not very secure about the future. Allowance should still be made for one recurrence of a depressive episode."

Not long after this, Santam's claim was settled for a very much reduced R176 000.

The ever doctor-friendly Medical Council wasted no time in granting all Lieberthal's requests. It would have been nice if complaints from patients got such prompt and favorable attention.

Toward the end of 1992, Prinsloo wrote to Dr. de Miranda to tell him that the President of the Medical Council had agreed to amend Lieberthal's conditions of practice to allow him to become a registrar under the supervision of Professor Erken. The Professor would then have to submit three-monthly reports to the Council. By that time, Lieberthal had already started the job.

He had to continue having psychiatric treatment from Dr. de Miranda, who would also be required to submit reports on his progress every three months. In addition, he was required to undertake random urine tests under the direction of Professor Erken.

Despite his dodgy background, the President still agreed to let him prescribe and administer all those high scheduled drugs.

Later, when Time Life inquired about Lieberthal's medical history in relation to a claim he had made, Prinsloo replied in a letter that Lieberthal's conditions of practice changed in September 1993. From then onwards, he still had to work as a registrar under Professor Erken, but the Council now only required annual reports from the Professor. De Miranda's reports on Lieberthal's follow-up treatment were extended to six-monthly intervals.

Lieberthal's reform was considered sufficient to allow him to treat private patients. On the recommendation of Professor Erken, he would be allowed to "participate in the scheme for limited private practice for registrars within the hospital set-up."

Chapter 4

Money, The Root Of All Evil

Lieberthal was put under severe financial strain when his partners in the Lyndhurst practice chucked him out without a cent. Even the year after that, his total earnings of R135 000 as the manager of the Rosebank Clinic did not do much to replenish his coffers.

The result was that when he started his second GP practice, the high living GP soon found himself deep in debt. His only way out was to be voluntarily sequestrated later that year.

In his handwritten Statement of Affairs lodged at the office of the Master of the Supreme Court in Pretoria, he gave details of his downfall. He blamed his insolvency on the fact that he had been in hospital for two of the five months that his new practice had been in existence. While he was away, he had employed a locum.

Giving another slant to the general practice he started in Lyndhurst in 1985, Lieberthal stated: "It grew rapidly beyond my wildest expectations. After one year, I had to double the size of my premises and take on a partner. It continued to grow to such an extent that my partner and I took on a third partner and we moved into Lyndhurst Clinic, which was designed and planned by myself. It was privately funded by an outside investor and we partners had the first opportunity to purchase it after five years. At that stage, I was riding on the crest of the wave with a very good income and I had the satisfaction of knowing that I had probably the biggest practice in Johannesburg."

This was not to last. In 1988, his initial partner Dr. Willies committed suicide, and this was to "tear me up emotionally up to this day". The size of the practice necessitated a third partner and his entry was "a disaster". He was clearly referring to Feinberg.

Patients did not readily want to see his junior partners. This resulted in him having an enormous patient load which caused him persistent stress and physical symptoms of headaches, irritability, insomnia, and the like. "By the end of 1989, I realized I could not spend a single day longer in that practice. I had to make a career change."

When his first back operation failed after his second car accident, he spent the next five months on "strong, habit-forming analgesics; being hospitalized and rehabilitated". Another operation was necessary, and he was once again placed on strong habit forming pain killers.

His financial problems increased when he went into private practice for the second time after being unable to meet his commitments on the salary of a hospital manager.

"On reflection, I realize that despite the circumstances, I continued to live at my same standard of living. I constantly reassured myself, irrationally, that once my practice started thriving, I would be able to meet my financial commitments."

He had "virtually no lucid recall of that dreadful time" when he was on drugs, and he was now trying to pick up the pieces of his life. He suffered a further setback because x-rays of his spine showed that one of the rods had broken and his fusion had failed to unite. "This will necessitate a redo operation," he added.

Lieberthal had assets in the form of properties in Norwood and Houghton Estate; household effects; motor vehicles, medical equipment, and debtors valued at R1 146 300. His liabilities to various banks, on the other hand, totaled R2 738 357, making a deficiency of R1 592 057.

What his trustee, Selwyn Trakman, discovered was extremely damning. Certain banks informed him that they held security for their claims by virtue of them having entered installment sale agreements with the insolvent.

"It now transpires that the assets that form the subject of these agreements were fictitious and that these aggrieved creditors may well elect to institute proceedings against the insolvent," Trakman informed creditors.

Among Lieberthal's debts were R48 296 owed to Allied Bank for medical and office equipment; R200 215 to Investec Bank for paintings, and R29 878 to Wesbank for a computer. The reality was the medical and office equipment were not even worth half of what he owed. There were no paintings, and the computer was worth a mere R300.

Hardly surprisingly, the doctor was unwilling or unable to produce records of his affairs.

In August 1992, Trakman told the Master of the Supreme Court that he believed the estate had a claim of R100 000 against an insurer for a car that was stolen prior to sequestration. "Correspondence with the insurer has elicited a response that they repudiate liability on, what we consider to be spurious grounds."

He wanted to sue the insurer. To do this, he got the Master's permission to employ an attorney and counsel. He needed them to do the necessary cross-examining of the insurer's representative to get him to explain why the claim had been repudiated.

Seven months later, a hearing was held at the Johannesburg Magistrate's Court before Henna Raath. The evidence presented proved that the grounds for repudiation were not as "spurious" as Trakman had first believed.

The spotlight was once again put on Lieberthal's lack of morality when it came to making insurance claims, which he seemed to have regarded as a source of easy money.

Evidence was given that not only had the car not been stolen. There was also considerable doubt as to whether there had been an alarm system and radio in the 1971 Mercedes Benz 280 SL. It was still subject to a hire purchase agreement in the name Mr. T.E. Rabi, the man Lieberthal claimed to have bought it from for R100 000. And the purchase was believed to be "false" as Lieberthal could not prove this.

Lieberthal's claims for the car and what was in it were repudiated under the clause in the policy that stated: "If any claim in any way seems fraudulent or if any fraudulent mode or method by the insured or any other person acting on his behalf is used to benefit him, all benefits of this policy will be annulled."

The Magistrate summed up the situation by saying, "It is clear that various criminals committed various crimes, or the possibility exists that various crimes have been committed, either by the person in whose name it was done, or by the insolvent, or by the supplier, and I now wish to refer the case to the Attorney-General for prosecution."

In 1996, Lieberthal successfully applied to the Supreme Court in Johannesburg to be rehabilitated because he intended to start his own practice as a spinal surgeon in October of that year.

He was effectively cleared when Trakman reported to the Master that he did not know of anything which would justify the Court in refusing the insolvent's rehabilitation. This was in spite of the fact that, in dealing with the estate, he found Lieberthal had not complied with certain aspects of the Insolvency Act relating to things like keeping proper accounts. These were in addition to Lieberthal's attempt to defraud the insurance company, as well as the fictitious goods that were financed.

So, as if someone had waved a magic wand, all these offences disappeared when he was rehabilitated. All his medical restrictions had also evidently been lifted.

He soon had a lot of patients with a variety of back and neck disorders coming to see him full of hope for a cure, unaware of his questionable background or what his treatment might have in store for them.

Had our physician learnt his lesson from these narrow escapes, or was he going to just shrug them off as unjustified attacks on his unblemished character?

Time would reveal a most disturbing picture.

Chapter 5

Dread Disease

Not content with making dubious insurance claims for his back injuries, Wynne Lieberthal, his relatives, and friends hit on another crafty money-making scheme that was going to solve all their financial woes. It had its dangers, but the prospect of instant riches made it very much worth the risk. Then, too, they were no doubt banking on that glow of respectability that generally surrounds doctors.

At that time, dread disease was a relatively new concept in life insurance. It enabled people who insured their lives to have additional cover for certain life-threatening illnesses such as cancer and heart disease. It meant that once the policy holder was diagnosed with one of the stipulated ailments, the amount for which they were insured under this section would be paid.

This was very appealing to a lot of people because they would get a substantial sum while they were still alive to help them with their recovery. It was even more appealing to Wynne and his bent broker. They saw another very sinister application for this kind of cover.

The conspirators consisted of Michael Masail, a life insurance broker and director of the Financial Workshop in Sandton, a very up market part of Johannesburg's Northern suburbs. Then there was Wynne himself; his twin brother Hugh; Hugh's wife, Janine; Bernard Markuschowitz, Hugh's onetime business partner and doctor, Attila Szabo.

The three Lieberthals, Markuschowitz, and Szabo took out dread disease policies through Masail. Steven Brower, a general practitioner friend of Dr. Lieberthal's, merely played a supporting role.

From 1991 to 1993, the five of them applied for policies with total life cover of R3.7-million complete with dread disease amounts totaling around R2.1-million split between various companies. In 1993, the companies woke up to the fact that there was something decidedly odd going on; something not at all in keeping with the generally held belief of how doctors should behave.

Professor Erken could not have known that the enterprise of two of his students had extended to a type of operating procedure that was never part of the Medical School's curriculum. Szabo was also a student there, and that's probably where he and Lieberthal teamed up.

The policies had only recently been issued when cancer suddenly broke out among the group as if it had become a contagious disease.

That was when I was called in to investigate the claims that had been coming in. A former investigative journalist on The Star, a daily newspaper in Johannesburg and The Sunday Times, the country's largest selling Sunday paper, I had been a private eye specializing in life insurance for some years.

In the three-year period Wynne took policies with Fedlife, Time Life, and Liberty Life. The basic life cover totaled R1.4-million with R550 000 on the dread disease side.

Dr. "Mossie" Nathan was the GP who did an insurance medical examination on his fellow doctor for Fedlife in October 1991. It was to establish that Wynne's health was up to the standard required before a policy could be issued. The form Dr. Nathan completed, which was pretty standard in the industry, consisted not only of his findings but also the answers Wynne gave about his previous medical history.

In the medical questionnaire Wynne signed, he never mentioned his drug abuse. He answered "No" to just about every question, including the one that asked: "If not already stated, have you during the past five years been hospitalized, taken any sedatives or drugs for medical or other reasons, or consulted any doctor including regular general check-ups."

He did mention his 1983 and 1990 back operations which necessitated him having to answer questions in an additional Back Questionnaire. In this, he claimed to have been pain-free since his 1990 operation. The dozy staff at Fedlife never questioned how he could he could have had a back operation in 1990 without being in hospital.

Wynne was also asked if he still participated in sport and he wrote: "Yes, jogging, squash and gym." On the face of it he was hale and hearty, over all his backache completely. At the bottom of the form, just above his signature, it stated: "I hereby declare that the above particulars and answers are complete and true."

But were they?

He again conveniently failed to disclose anything about being treated for a drug problem in the Time Life application form completed in June 1992.

He had not yet finished accumulating policies. In May 1993, he took advantage of a special offer from Liberty Life. This type of policy was tailor-made for people up to no good because no medical examination was required. All he had to do was to satisfy the company that his most recent South African policy taken after May 1990 had been issued at standard rates after he had made a full medical declaration.

He named the Norwich Life policy he took in 1992. Dr. Nathan had also examined him on that occasion. I think this policy lapsed soon afterwards, possibly because he couldn't afford the premiums at that time.

Dr. Nathan would have been totally unaware of the lies Wynne was telling him about his medical background and nor would he have had any inkling that this was part of a well-planned insurance swindle.

In July 1993, it was time to start claiming instead of wasting more money on premiums.

Wynne's claims were based on a small growth, removed from the skin on the back of his neck by Dr. Szabo that they said was cancerous. I spoke to both Wynne and Szabo about this, and their stories were littered with inconsistencies when compared with the claim and medical forms that were submitted.

Szabo completed medical reports for all the companies.

He was an inexperienced 30-year-old doctor from Hungary who had only been in South Africa a short while. Handsome, with a mop of dark hair, he looked the part of the dashing surgeon. He would particularly impress his lady patients, of that I had no doubt.

I saw Szabo at his flat in Corlett Gardens in Johannesburg. He said he operated on Wynne in the casualty department of the Johannesburg Hospital because that was the hospital where Wynne was working. His reason for not completing any records there was that he was not attached to that hospital.

Szabo sent the specimen he had taken from Wynne to the hospital's laboratory. When I went there, the pieces of the puzzled began to show a picture that nobody would have been happy to hang on the wall at the Wits Medical School. Wynne and Szabo not only trained there, but they also submitted papers jointly at several congresses of the South African Orthopaedic Association.

There I spoke to Dr. Ronnie Cohen, whose name appeared at the bottom of the laboratory's findings that described the specimen as a "skin ellipse that was a superficial spreading, malignant melanoma." Cohen got the slide out and had another look at it under the microscope.

"There seems to have been a mistake on the report," he said solemnly. "The maximum depth of the invasion has been put down as 8.5 millimeters. I have never seen a tumor of this kind that was that deep. The measurement should have been 0.85 millimeters. We normally deal with them in the following categories, less than 0.75 millimeters; 0.76 millimeters to 1.5 millimeters and then above 1.5 millimeters.

"If a doctor got a report that a tumor like this had gone to a depth of 8.5 millimeters it would mean a virtual death sentence. That's why I am surprised that Dr. Lieberthal never came back to me to query this."

The diameter of the tumor was correct. "It was a big one which would have been around for years because tumors of this kind don't grow that fast. That's why I would have expected Dr. Lieberthal to have noticed it a lot earlier and done something about it."

Questioned further, Szabo showed an alarming lack of knowledge for somebody who was happy to remove a growth of this size out of a fellow doctor's neck.

"Can you interpret lab reports?" I asked.

"The report gave the depth of the tumor as 8.5 millimeters. Does this indicate how bad it was?"

"No, it doesn't. I was happy with the accuracy of the report."

"Do you know that Dr. Cohen at the lab told me he had never come across a tumor of this kind that was 8.5 millimeters deep?" I said, knowing I had him stumped.

Flustered, he replied, "I don't know. I mean I can cut it out but I, I don't have the knowledge to compare it."

"In view of your inexperience, why did he get you to do this when he could have got a top surgeon to do it for nothing?"

"Because, I mean, it didn't look so bad."

I showed him the Time Life medical report he completed for the claim. "You stated here that further treatment would depend on subsequent tests." I spat the words out in a tone that sent a clear message that I was determined to get the truth out of him.

"*Ja*, Wynne told me that."

Surprised, I replied, "Oh, Wynne told you that?"

"Yes. And, I mean, we discussed it and we saw that, ah, we excised it in healthy tissue. You can't really do more. I mean you can do some blood tests, but they usually don't say anything."

"You mentioned there that one possible treatment was chemotherapy?" I pointed out.

"*Ja*, if you find something in the blood." But he didn't think any blood tests had been done.

"In the report you did for Time Life, you stated you first saw Dr. Lieberthal for this condition on the 26th of June 1993 and that the condition started in 'mid-June 1993'," I said expecting more bunkum.

"You see, I never saw that before. It was somewhere in the hair."

"But, in the Fedlife report, you stated Dr. Lieberthal only became aware of this possibly cancerous condition on the 26th. So, there's a clash of facts."

"I don't know. I can't remember what date we excised that thing."

"In the Liberty Life report, you wrote that you first saw him on the 26th of June and again on the 29th. For the 26th, you put 'Dg, ulcerated pigment lesion'."

"That was the diagnosis."

"Then for the 29th of June, you wrote 'treatment'. Is that when you excised it?" I asked, wondering when he was going to realize that his answers were getting him deeper and deeper into a very unsavory affair that could bring his medical career to an untimely end.

"Looks like it," he replied. "You see, I can't remember exactly when this was done."

"Okay. Then you say that on the 29th 'histology confirms melanoma'. But this lab report here says 'Date taken 29/6; date received 29/6; date reported 5/7/93'. How did you know on the 29th that the histology had confirmed melanoma?"

"I don't know."

When I spoke to Wynne, he said he had an ulcer on the back of his neck. He drew a circle about the size of a pea on a piece of paper to show me what size it was. "I only became aware of it possibly a couple of days before it was removed."

Revealing my ace, but hoping he would not recognize it as one, I said, "You saw that the lab report gave the depth of the tumor as 8.5 millimeters. Were you satisfied that this was correct?"

"*Ja*, I had no reason not to think, so especially as they said, 'deep and lateral margins are well clear of malignancy'. You know, I was obviously happy that the whole thing had been removed."

Was he as ignorant about these things as Szabo, or was he just assuming that I would not know any better?

At the end of the Time Life document, Wynne "solemnly" declared "that to the best of my knowledge all the information in this report is accurate and complete and I have not withheld any information which could influence a decision on this claim".

He could not have told a bigger whopper than that, was what they might have said to him had he still been at school.

And the whoppers didn't end there. At the end of the Fedlife claim form, he declared that: "I am solvent and my estate has not been sequestrated."

When I asked him about this, he confessed, "You know it's not correct."

He put the blame on Dr. Nathan for the omission of his drug problem. He told the doctor about it, he claimed, "He didn't put it down, but I have to concede I signed the documents where it does not, in fact, say that I have had, um, rehabilitation for an addiction of analgesics. I'm not proud of it and it's not something I want to talk about."

Predictably, Dr. Nathan denied being told about this.

Another odd aspect of the Fedlife policy was that it did not belong to Wynne. The owner was Masail, the broker. He wrote in the application form that he was Dr. Lieberthal's friend and the policy had been taken as security for a loan.

Wynne was vague when I asked him why Masail was the owner of this policy. "I assume that policy was taken at a time when I had no financial resources. Mike may have paid a couple of premiums, but I paid the majority of them."

According to Feinberg, Masail used to be one of Wynne's patients when they were in practice together.

"Apparently Wynne owed him quite a bit of money," I said.

"Whether it's true or not, you'll never know," he replied. "When it came to Wynne, everybody owed him money."

Fedlife paid Masail R221 566 for Dr. Lieberthal's claim and Time Life handed out another R150 000 to Wynne himself. The doctor told me he accepted he did not tell these companies the truth, and that he was prepared to repay the money he got, but I doubt that this ever happened in view of the move that Masail subsequently made.

This meant that in a ten-year period, Wynne's insurance bonanza had netted him almost a million rand. A tidy little sum, considering all he had to do was to convince insurance companies that seemed keener to part with their money than to repudiate a dubious claim. A reputation for not paying claims was bad for business, especially if you were one of the small fry firms competing against the whales of the industry.

Being one of the whales, it was not surprising that Liberty Life was the exception: It was a lot shrewder. Its claims department did a proper background check. Wynne's R200 000 claim was repudiated. In a letter signed by Gavin Came, Liberty's deputy general manager in charge of individual business, Wynne was told that he had not qualified for the Special Offer because he failed to tell Norwich Life about his drug problem.

Came concluded his letter by saying: "You warranted the truth and accuracy of all information supplied by yourself and agreed that, should any material fact be withheld or misstated, the contract may be declared void and all monies paid into the contract forfeited. In view of the circumstances referred to above, the contract is declared void and hereby cancelled."

That was the second insurance company that had caught him telling lies. And Dr. Lieberthal's career as a fully fledged surgeon had not yet started.

Unfortunately, both Fedlife and Time Life had been unaware of Wynne's deceit when they settled. The payments were made before I began my investigation at the instigation of Standard General, a company that was involved with some of the other members of the Gang.

In November 1993, Paul Sieberhagen, an advocate who was head of Fedlife's legal services, wrote a letter to Masail regarding Wynne's dread disease claim. They had paid Masail R221 566 in July 1993, and they wanted the money back from him as he was the owner of the policy.

He described the non-disclosure about Dr. Lieberthal's drug dependency as being very material to the risk. "Had the fact been disclosed at the time of application, we would have declined to offer any terms. Similarly, had we been aware of this information at the time of the claim, we would have repudiated it."

A few days later, Masail replied on a Financial Workshop letterhead, which gave the firm's motto as "Building Security For You". He took the policy on

Dr. Lieberthal's life, he wrote, as security for the money the doctor owed him. In March 1993, Wynne had repaid the debt and was given the proceeds of the claim.

That did not satisfy Sieberhagen. He told Masail that, as he had been paid the money as the owner of the policy, he had to repay it and not Dr. Lieberthal. "We therefore urgently request you to return the claim proceeds to us to avoid the necessity of having to take further action."

In January 1994, a meeting was held in Fedlife's offices in central Johannesburg between Masail; Sieberhagen; Dr. Brennan Nelson the firm's financial strategist, and Darryl Morris, an outside legal adviser. Masail was told they felt that Dr. Lieberthal's claim was not a valid one.

"And we would like the bucks back," said Sieberhagen sternly.

"Okay," Masail replied, being surprisingly submissive. "Let me admit guilt where guilt is needed. Yes, I did help him non-disclose. He'd been a good friend of mine for a long time. I mean, I'm not going to deny it because there's no point. You know I did it and I know I did it. If we are going to talk openly, let's do it cards on the table."

The men listening had no idea at that stage why the glib-talking broker was making this remarkable confession with hardly any prompting. They were to find out soon enough that, although they might have thought they had the whip hand, Masail had a master plan that was soon to trump them all.

"At least that way I can show a little bit of good faith with you people," the broker's disclosure went on. "I thought, I thought, you know, thirty years down the line when there was a claim it wouldn't have made any difference anyhow that I'm guilty. Being a material nondisclosure, it's not a valid claim but I still think the growth is genuine."

"In other words, you believed the disease existed?" said Sieberhagen, who must have felt like a Catholic father in the confessional.

"I can't believe otherwise. Otherwise, I've got to start looking at my friends and saying, 'Hey guys, what are you doing to me?' You want your money back. I don't think you care if you get it back from Harry Oppenheimer, from me, or from Lieberthal. You want your funds back. Is that correct?"

"*Ja*, well, legally, we want it from you because the contract was with you," Sieberhagen told him.

Masail followed with a neat con man's tactic to buy time. "I'm bringing some money back from London," he continued with a sly grin. "I've got a small inheritance there that will more than cover this. It's going to take approximately forty-five days to get it here because it's on thirty day call. It's legal money. Are you prepared to give me the forty-five days? The total is a hundred and twenty-seven thousand pounds. Multiply that by five and I will have six hundred thousand rand. I think that will cover you guys quite adequately. I'll pay you what I owe you by the end of next month. If I don't pay you, you'll press criminal charges."

"It's an option, yes."

"I mean, let's be honest with each other. If I sort you out, will you drop the whole thing and forget about it? Will that be alright?"

Reluctant to accede to everything Masail was asking Sieberhagen refused to give such an undertaking unless Masail paid up.

Masail had been hospitalized on four occasions in the previous year, and that was why he had not got around to ceding the policy back to Wynne after he had been repaid, he claimed. "I wish I had because then it would have been out of my hands," he told his audience.

The broker had just come back from holiday and he assured his listeners he was "not running away." He needed to regain his credibility. "I've seen the error of my ways. This non-disclosure was the worst thing I ever did. But I'll be okay in the industry because I won't do it again, that you can be sure of."

His record went back to 1986 when he was with Southern Life. "I worked for them for eight years and during that time I wrote sixteen or eighteen thousand policies, and may be three or four of them were bum like this one. In this industry, it's not a bad record. But people forget everything that's good and remember all that's bad. Yes, I feel guilty for what I've done. Okay, I'll admit it in a closed room."

It was agreed that the necessary documents would be drawn up and they would meet again the following week. "I'll get my attorney to look at them to see there's nothing that really, ah, puts a knife in me because I must protect myself, more from the Lieberthal side than the Fedlife side," Masail said as he got up to leave. "If my attorney gives approval, then I'll sign."

Walking out of the building, he was probably congratulating himself on how well he had pulled it off. Not only had he succeeded in getting claims paid, but he had just completed the swindle with his best confidence trick of all.

Chapter 6

Wynne's Twin Joins In

Hugh Lieberthal, the doctor's twin brother, also had to be included in this insurance money-spinner. His Crusader Life policy began in March 1992. It was another one of those special offers which gave him life cover of R200 000 and dread disease cover of R100 000. In October of that year, he took another policy with Old Mutual that had basic life cover of R330 000 and R200 000 worth of dread disease insurance. So he was well set up.

Originality was not their strong point. When Hugh started claiming in April 1993, he, like his brother, also had a malignant melanoma.

Hugh's growth had been removed from his left calf by Dr. Brower. His surgery was in Turffontein, a relatively poor area in the southern part of Johannesburg, whereas Hugh lived kilometers away in the more affluent suburb of Linksfield on the other side of the city. Nobody would have expected anybody in a posh area like Linksfield to go to an ordinary GP in Turffontein for this kind of procedure unless he had some very unusual talent which was not available elsewhere.

As was the case with Wynne's cancer, the insurance companies were given an equally conflicting and confusing story as to what happened when Hugh's malignant growth occurred.

In the Old Mutual medical form Brower completed for the claim, he wrote that Hugh had first consulted him about what he described as the "dread disease" on 21 March 1993. He last saw him in relation to this two days later. In a similar form he filled in for Crusader on the same day, he came up with some new information. In the middle of January 1993, Hugh had what Brower called a "traumatic amputation mole" and his left calf was "sutured". He went on to state that he saw him again on "21-22/3/93" for "wide excision? Melanoma left calf".

The report by the Randburg laboratory of Doctors Gritzman, Thatcher, and Lewis described the specimen as a "pigmented skin lesion" with a "central surgical" scar. This indicated that there had been an earlier operation at the same spot. It was diagnosed as being a malignant melanoma around an area of scaring and that the "tumor extended up to both lateral excision lines".

A specialist told me that you could not be certain all the cancer had been removed because ideally the specimen should have had a clear area all around it. The wise thing to have done in this case would have been to make a much wider cut and get another laboratory report to make sure that the excision lines were well clear of the malignancy. But nothing like that was done, at least not before the claims were submitted and probably at no stage after that.

In an effort to clarify what had happened, I spoke to Brower at his surgery. He appeared as nervous as a patient being prepared for their first big operation. At times, he gave the impression he was stuttering because a lot of his answers were full of ums and ahs and words that were repeated, sometimes as many as three times in succession.

He said the "hard" tumor on Hugh's left calf that he removed had evolved. "This means part of it had broken off," he explained helpfully in layman's terms for me. "It was oozing and, um, at that stage, I thought it looks like a melanoma. The next day we, um, excised that, okay."

"How deep did you have to cut him?" I asked.

"You've got to do quite a, quite a… a… you've got to go clear of the border. It was a quite longish, longish cut." He had evidently kept his records to a minimum, judging by what he said next. "Again, I never write down sizes of things."

The operation was done in his rooms because that was the easiest place to do it and the growth was not in a "problem area". Determined to keep him talking, I asked him what he had advised Hugh to do after he had received the verdict from the laboratory.

With the same hesitant speech, he continued, "Okay, he basically required um… um… um… because normally what you do, you advise them to… to seek specialist advice, okay. And um….."

"But did you advise him to do that?" I asked, trying to get a more definite answer.

"*Ja, ja, ja* he needs wide excision. But sometimes you can do one of two things with a melanoma. Either you can, you can leave it, okay, which may be not the best thing medically to do or you must, you must do a wide excision. You know you must then go to see a surgeon."

"To your knowledge, was that done?"

"If something was done, I'm not sure because I don't have a follow up from the specialist. So I presume… either if he went to a specialist I wasn't informed or he left it as is."

"Wouldn't it be very dangerous to leave it as is?" I said, putting him on the spot.

"Mm, you see, we removed the whole tumor."

Fortunately, I had done enough research to know that what he had just told me was not supported by the evidence. So I asked, "But doesn't the lab report make it clear that you possibly didn't remove the whole tumor?"

"'Tumor extending up to both lateral lines of excision'," he read from the report. "Oh, that was to be, um, to be adequate, I would, I would imagine. But the point really is, *ja*, ideally he needs specialist care, surgical care."

It was all very airy-fairy with a lot to be desired when one considered that he had been treating one of man's most feared diseases. And when I again suggested that the lab report indicated he might not have removed the whole growth, he replied casually, "Oh, they, they might have meant that."

I was very tempted to up the tempo of my interrogation. But I had found from past experience that life companies tended to treat doctors with a lot of undue respect, in many cases. If they complained about the way an investigator had spoken to them, he often got told off, even if it was completely unjustified. I asked Brower if he had cut anything out of the same spot on Hugh's leg on a previous occasion.

"No," he said.

"Nobody had?"

"Not to my knowledge. I hadn't treated him."

"What I mean is, you saw no evidence of that?"

"No".

What he had just told me conflicted with what he wrote in the Crusader Life medical certificate. I would have thought that had he done what he described as a "traumatic amputation mole" on Hugh's left calf in mid-January 1993, it would have been sent to a laboratory for a report. Or was he just saying this to explain the report on the specimen taken in March, which indicated that it had a previous surgical scar across it?

I spoke to Hugh Lieberthal at his home eight months after the growth was supposed to have been removed from his leg. Far from clearing up the confusion, he made it worse.

"How did you discover this problem?" I asked.

"I scratched my leg, and it started bleeding."

"You mean scratched it with your …"

Without even giving me a chance to complete the question, he answered quickly, "No, no, on a wall."

That was a new version which he had not informed Dr. Brower about because the doctor wrote in the Crusader medical certificate that it had not been caused by an injury.

"It started bleeding, and I went to see Dr. Brower," he continued, unaware of how he was white-anting his own claim. "He took it out, and a few days later, I went to see him again to make sure everything was okay. Then he told me it was malignant, and I needed to come back again in another few days. That's when he took the stitches out."

"Did he suggest you have any further treatment?"

"Look, it's okay from what I understand it. It's clear at the edges where he took it out." In an effort to get my sympathy, he added, "Okay. I've not told my wife about this. The reason is quite simple. In January, her mother had a third of her lung removed, and because of so much trauma, I just felt that it wasn't worth telling her. There's enough that a person can, you know, handle, okay? What I did decide to do, um, I decided on an annual basis to go and have a checkup. I've been fine since then, there's been no problems."

His brother had arranged for him to see Brower. They knew each other because they were at medical school together.

He agreed he had seen the laboratory report, which I showed him. I told him that where it stated "tumor extending up to both lateral excision lines" it meant that the tumor was right up to the edge of the specimen and might not have been removed completely.

"That's not how it was explained to me," he replied, showing no sign of concern. "I was told that it goes to the edges, but as it does not go over the edges, it's clear. You got me a little bit worried there. If that is what you're saying, I most certainly will go and find out first thing on Monday morning. I'm most happy to go and see a surgeon about it, absolutely. I mean, I understand now. I don't know what your medical background is."

"I don't have any," I told him, "but I've spoken to specialists."

"Well, I have it how it was explained to me and obviously it wasn't explained very well".

"Have you ever had any problems before this?"

"In what regard?"

"Lumps being taken out of you?"

"No."

Three months after I had first spoken to Hugh, he told me he had arranged to see Dr. Philip Steyn, a general surgeon at Mulbarton private hospital. He did not keep his initial appointment, but he finally saw Dr. Steyn in March 1994, a year after the so-called cancerous growth was removed from his leg.

Earlier, I had sent a letter to Dr. Steyn telling him about the investigation I was doing. I asked if he could tell me if Hugh had previously had some kind of growth removed from the same spot, and if he could throw any light on why Hugh was only now seeking a specialist's advice. He chose not to answer me specifically. All he did was to send me a copy of his report that he had sent to Dr. Brower.

The significant part about it was that he was told that, "a pigmented skin lesion had been excised from the same site a number of years ago. He (Hugh) was uncertain what the histology of the first lesion had been." So the stories kept changing.

Dr. Steyn ended his letter by stating: "There is no evidence of any recurrence at present. Because of the histology report that the tumor was extending up to the line of the excision, I have advised a wider excision of the scar. He must also then be followed up more closely in order to detect any recurrence early."

I do not believe that Hugh had the additional operation that Dr. Steyn recommended. He already knew what the true position was.

On one occasion that I saw Dr. Lieberthal, I asked, "How's your brother now?"

"He's okay." He made out that, as the two of them were twins, their cancer was hereditary.

"What treatment is he having?"

"There is not much one can do there. It depends obviously where the site of the lesion is." He was talking as if he was referring to some anonymous person. "If it's on a limb, you can isolate the flow of blood. Then chemotherapy can be given into the limb and, in theory, it will knock off any cells that would spread from the melanoma to other parts of the body. But this is very sort of theoretical, without, it's without any kind of solid basis behind it."

"Has he had that done?"

"Oh no, the value of that is far from being established. It's a very new phenomenon, you know, I think the margins of the specimen were clear and he's hoping for the best."

Hugh's Old Mutual claim was paid, as well as the Crusader one, even though that company was in some kind of difficulty, making a total of R300 000. Again, these payments were made before I came on the scene.

Flushed with success, Wynne and his accomplices must have felt they had hit a winning streak with gullible companies making out check after check. They were certainly not going to stop now.

Chapter 7

The Scheme

Never short of an idea to boost business, Masail set up the Double Jay Group Scheme through Time Life for employees of Hugh Lieberthal's Double Jay printing firm. It was a dubious plan that had Time Life totally blinded by the prospect of enabling this small company to get well in with a powerful brokerage. When it began in August 1992, it offered only life cover. According to the list submitted to the insurance company, there were nine employees including Hugh Lieberthal and his 36-year-old wife, Janine. All of them had their lives covered for R250 000 and they were said to have joined the firm at the beginning of 1991, when the business began.

Hugh ran Double Jay from his home in Linksfield. This was where the printing was done, and he also had a stall at the Bruma Lake Flea Market.

From its inception, the Group Scheme was a disaster because the total monthly premium of R450 for life cover amounting to R1 478 000 was not paid with any regularity. Time Life often sent letters to Masail complaining that premiums were in arrears. Odd payments were made either by Double Jay or, inexplicably, out of Masail's trust account. Ironically, Time Life bragged on its letterhead that it was a "Non-listed Award Finalist, 1992."

A Time Life internal memorandum that was given to me made me wonder what I was seeing. After the Scheme's appalling payment record, this company was still serious about carrying on with it and making it still more attractive.

On 1 August 1993, the Scheme began all over again. This time it had dread disease cover added to the life insurance. As it was a group scheme, no employee had to give any kind of undertaking that they were in good health. It was also made even more of a bargain because a continuation option was included. All those who left the Scheme could take individual policies with Time Life without having to answer any medical questions.

By this time, the number of employees had almost doubled to sixteen. Three of the original nine had disappeared and the additional names included Dr. Wynne Lieberthal, his wife Deborah, and Markuschowitz.

The total monthly premium was now R1 850. If Double Jay and Masail between them could not pay the original premium of R450 timeously, how did anybody in the employee benefits department think that they would be able to come up with the new payment? Not surprisingly, the shocking payment pattern continued. Time Life received Hugh Lieberthal's personal check for R973 in August, well short of what the first premium should have been. The following month, R1 850 was paid from Masail's trust account. Nobody at the insurance company seemed to think it was odd that now no money was being received from Double Jay itself.

According to the rules of the Scheme, a member had to be an employee or a full-time working director in the permanent service of Double Jay Printing. "Service" was defined as somebody who was actively employed by Double Jay for not less than twenty hours per week. Suddenly Wynne Lieberthal, the doctor who was training to become an orthopedic surgeon, and his 34-year-old wife, were working for a printing firm. He received commission, he told me, if he introduced somebody who needed printing, but he was not on the staff.

His wife had evidently changed or added to the jobs she did because, in March 1992, Lieberthal told Donaldson that his industrious spouse, who was a qualified nursing sister, worked part-time doing home nursing, post-natal work, debt collecting, and she also worked one night a week at the Rosebank Clinic. At that stage, they had a daughter aged seven and two sons aged five and three. He described his wife Debbie "as a strong driving force in their marriage and that honesty and integrity are very important to her".

A Time Life new entrant schedule for the Scheme signed in August 1993 by Hugh listed both Masail and Wynne Lieberthal as being among the members. Everyone on the Scheme was said to have been at work at Double Jay on the first day of their membership, which was given as the 1st of August 1993. It did not occur to these con-men that this was a Sunday.

In September 1993, Hugh wrote a letter to Time Life on a Double Jay letterhead saying that the business was being sold and so the Scheme ceased at the end of that month.

The ink on Hugh's signature on that letter was hardly dry before Masail was getting people to sign new Time Life application forms to enable them to be covered under the continuation option. No matter how sick they were, they were guaranteed to get a policy. They were Masail, Wynne's wife Deborah, Markuschowitz, and four others who were clearly not privy to the fraudulent aspect of what was going on. Most of them got dread disease cover of R150 000 with some of them getting slightly less. Their life insurance ranged between R206 000 to R50 000 for those who presumably could not afford higher premiums.

In addition to members of the Gang, the others had also been Masail's clients. The majority of them had such a poor medical history, they would never have been able to get dread disease cover normally. Some of them had never heard of Double Jay, while the nearest others had got to working for this firm was trying to get printing orders at Masail's request.

The Scheme was clearly another fraud, and Time Life turned out to be the perfect firm to dupe. I could not establish who at this company had been directly responsible for approving it. I wouldn't have blamed anybody there if they had wanted to distance themselves from it.

When I saw Hugh about his claims, I also spoke to him about Double Jay Printing. He said he was the sole proprietor.

Markuschowitz began working with him at Double Jay. Earlier in that same year, they started another business together in nearby Glenhazel called Design Print.

"We ran it for four or five months together," Hugh said. "We then dissolved the partnership very amicably, and he's still consulting to me on Macintosh computers." Markuschowitz carried on with the Design Print business on his own.

Masail undertook to arrange the Scheme and employ people to do sales for the printing business.

He had always relied on Masail to deal with his insurance matters, and he had never had any problems. "I still don't have a problem with him. I'm not disputing that my signature is there. I told you right from the beginning I don't know these people. The Scheme ran for about two months and there was no business forthcoming from these people, so I said to him, 'Mike, I'm not prepared to carry on'."

As soon as the scheme ceased, Hugh Lieberthal's wife, Janine, took a policy under the continuation option. It gave her cover of R250 000 for her life and R150 000 for dread disease.

Just thirteen days later, she submitted a claim for R150 000. A medical certificate dated 27 September 1993 and completed by her brother-in-law Dr. Lieberthal, was produced with a laboratory report confirming breast cancer.

According to him, he had known his sister-in-law for thirteen years. He first treated her in 1982 for minor ailments and, for the next 11 years, she had no need of a doctor. That was what Wynne expected Time Life to believe because she next consulted him in 1993 for migraine and sinusitis. The cancer was discovered later the same year. In the "Cancer" section of the certificate, Wynne continued to dramatize Janine's illness. Asked where the site and the extent of the growth was Lieberthal wrote: "Unstaged at present but probably metastatic." The spread of a primary tumor to other parts of the body is when it becomes metastatic and staging is a series of tests that may be done to establish just how far the disease has progressed.

Asked in the form whether it was malignant or non-malignant he wrote: "Malignant + +."

The report confirming cancer that Dr. Lieberthal produced with the Time Life medical certificate he completed came from the well-known and long established laboratory of Dr. Piet van Drimmelen and Partners. On 22

September 1993, they received five milliliters of clear fluid taken from the right breast of a 37-year-old female patient. It was diagnosed as "Malignant duct epithelial cells in keeping with derivation from a duct carcinoma."

The validity of this could not be doubted. But the laboratory had no way of knowing where the specimen had come from. For that, it had to rely on the word of a doctor who had already proved that telling the truth was far from being one of his strongest points.

When I spoke to Dr. Lieberthal in November 1993, he told me he had done a "needle aspiration" on his sister-in-law. This involved putting a needle into her breast and drawing out a sample of fluid.

He was vague when asked what further treatment she had: "I don't know, you know. Um, she, she has got a bit of an emotional problem and she has been delaying and dilly dallying. She's apparently discussed the matter with her gynecologist and, um, she's been advised to have further treatment."

"By who?"

"By a specialist."

"*Ja*, but which specialist?"

"That's for her to decide. I'm the GP. I don't make those decisions."

"But didn't you send her to a specialist?"

"She didn't want to go. She didn't want to go." He made out that this was because her mother had part of a lung removed and Janine could not face having cancer herself.

In Section 1 of the medical certificate, Dr. Lieberthal was asked: "Is there anything noteworthy, or with which Time Life should be made acquainted, in the history, progress or treatment of the case?"

His misleading answer was: "No."

With the help of Dr. Lieberthal, Masail was now increasing the pressure on Time Life to have Janine's claim paid. The two of them took the unusual step of going to the Norwood Police station where they had affidavits signed in front of a Commissioner of Oaths. They both swore that Janine had no previous history of cancer.

In all my experience of doing life insurance investigations, I had never come across anything like this before and nor had I ever seen such a blatant warning to the company that cried out: Watch, watch out, you are about to be taken for a very expensive ride if you choose to ignore this.

What were the claims assessors thinking at Time Life when Masail produced these two worthless bits of paper? Nobody there thought to ask Masail why Janine had not made a similar affidavit if her previous history was considered to be so relevant. The master minds were keeping her well out of the way. Evidently, they felt she was the weak link, not that their own performances were all that convincing.

In any event, as Janine's policy was an extension of the Double Jay Group Scheme, no medical evidence had been required when it was issued. There was absolutely no necessity for Masail and Lieberthal to go to such extraordinary lengths to try and convince the company that Janine had been cancer-free until her brother-in-law discovered she had the disease. They were protesting far, far too much.

Time Life's claim was reinsured through Mercantile and General Reinsurance in Cape Town. And, when Val Hardwick, their claims assessor, got the details from Time Life, she suggested that the claim should not be admitted at that stage and that Janine should be examined by Dr. Anthony Crosley, a physician specialist in Johannesburg.

Re-insurers for life companies can make suggestions as to how a claim should be dealt with, but the final decision always rests with the company itself. The result is that, every now and again, a farcical situation arises where the re-insurer's advice is ignored and the life company pays a decidedly dodgy claim. In these cases, the re-insurer may refuse to pay the re-insured portion depending on the relationship it has with the firm concerned, or the life insurer won't submit a claim to its re-insurer.

Time Life never wavered when it came to turning a blind eye to all the red flags the Masail camp kept unfurling all over the place. Hardwick's useful advice was ignored, and that cost R150 000, part or all of which her company might have had to pay. The money went to Masail because Janine signed a special power of attorney authorizing him to get it. The reason she gave was: "That I have already received the funds due to me."

I came on the scene too late to stop the payment. But what I dug up afterwards made Janine's claim look even more putrid than some of the others.

Even Time Life's managing director appeared to have realized too late what a mess they had made. This became clear when Masail was cajoled into signing a most peculiar letter. Instead of allaying the fears of those who felt the company had been cheated, it only fortified this perception.

The letter, witnessed by Bill Haslam, Time Life's MD and addressed to him, was a kind of backhanded confession. In it Masail made this empty promise: "This serves to indemnify Time Life against the above mentioned claim proving to be a non-claim in terms of the dread disease definition of cancer. Should this claim prove to be a non-claim I undertake to repay Time Life or its re-insurer the full amount of the claim valued at R150 000 over an agreed upon time period with interest thereon being calculated at the prime overdraft rate to its corporate clients as amended from time to time."

In August 1992, Janine had a mammogram done by Dr. Selwyn Strano at the Bagleyston Clinic in Norwood. By the time I went there, Strano had left South Africa and his radiology practice had been taken over by Dr. Harry Said.

The records showed Janine had no history of breast cancer and she had felt no lumps. The doctor concluded that there was no evidence of malignancy. She named her gynecologist as Dr. Mervyn Hurwitz, to whom the mammogram report was sent.

A year later, Janine saw Dr. Hurwitz for a checkup. He told me that he examined her breasts and found no lumps. "At the time Mrs. Lieberthal was not complaining about anything and as far as I was concerned, everything was fine."

About two weeks after Janine had seen her gynecologist, Lieberthal drew the controversial fluid from her right breast that was supposed to have revealed conclusively that she had cancer. When I told Dr. Hurwitz about this he said, "I'm flabbergasted. If she had been diagnosed as having cancer of the breast I would have expected her to come back to me. But I've heard nothing about this. Dr. Lieberthal's wife, who is due to have a baby soon, is also one of my patients and she has never mentioned anything about Mrs. Janine Lieberthal having cancer."

As a result of pressure from Mercantile and General, and possibly because of the interviews I had with Wynne and Hugh, Janine went to see Dr. John Tinker, a surgeon based at the Kenridge Hospital. The appointment was made by Mercantile and General. In a letter to Hardwick, Tinker wrote: "She consulted me, perhaps unaware of the communication from you in terms of her medical background. She brought an undated referring letter from Dr. Wynne Lieberthal giving the history detailed to me on your faxed report".

Having examining Janine, Tinker could find no evidence of cancer. "I informed her that I could not feel the lump or cyst which was aspirated in September 1993 and I suggested she have a mammogram. It would appear unlikely that she in fact has a carcinoma in her right breast with no palpable mass or mammographic evidence of a tumor after an interval of three months."

In February 1994, four months after Janine was diagnosed as having breast cancer, she finally had a mammogram. The result explained exactly why she had been so reluctant to go for this test. Tinker's findings were confirmed by Dr. Said when the mammogram again showed no sign of malignancy. I was given a copy of the form that was completed by one of the radiologists on the basis of answers given by Janine. The reason for the examination was given as "Routine," and Janine answered "No" to the one that asked, "Do you feel a lump?" The question, "History of breast cancer, self?" was not answered.

Just five days after Janine's second mammogram, I went to her home to try to get a firsthand account from her. As I started to speak to her, as she came out of her front door, her husband rushed out and ushered me into his office nearby.

"Can I see you first of all? Can you tell me what it's about, please?" he demanded.

After he had made it clear that he would not let me speak to his wife, I got to the real point of my visit.

"From what Dr. Tinker says, your wife has not got cancer," I said.

I would be delighted if that was the truth," he replied. "I mean, nobody wants to have cancer. We've got such a history of it in the family that is quite unbelievable."

"The question really remains, what's going to happen about the money that was paid to your wife?" I asked, knowing full well that Time Life was unlikely to get it back. In my experience, life companies that had been defrauded seldom went to court to recover their money. My impression was that they did not want to expose their incompetence or give potential clients the idea they might be sticky on claims.

"Well, I think that is a reasonable, a reasonably simple question to answer," Hugh replied, as if he had every intention of doing what he then proposed. "If that is the situation—and I'm saying a big 'if', okay—I will make arrangements with, with Time Life to have it repaid. I'm not, I'm not running away from my obligations. If that is the situation, then I'm quite sure that I will be able to come to some sort of an arrangement with them. You obviously would know if they would be willing to make an arrangement."

"You must appreciate that if your wife hasn't got cancer, they'd obviously like to get their money back."

"Sure. Paying it back in one lump sum, I mean that would be impossible. I've had various setbacks for which the money has been used. Um, be that as it may, if that is the situation then I'm quite happy to make an arrangement with them to repay the money. And if it's got to be repaid with interest, so be it. I'm not running away from them. To me, it's more important that my wife is well, than the money."

The money Hugh and his wife got didn't last long. In March 1995, she went insolvent, and he followed his brother's unenviable example a few months later.

Chapter 8

Spreading Cancer

Bernard Markuschowitz had two policies. The one was with Standard General and came into force in April 1993. It provided basic life cover of R200 000 and dread disease cover for the same amount. The other one was taken with Time Life in September 1993 under the Double Jay Scheme's continuation option. The cover he got here was for amounts that were the same as those from Standard General.

In his Standard General application, Markuschowitz, also known as Marks, claimed he was a director of his own company that designed computer systems. He had been in the same job for ten years and was earning a salary of R12 000 a month. It should have been more than enough for him to afford the premium of R355 a month. This was supposed to be paid out of his Natal Building Society transmission account.

The first time the account was debited without success. The following day, Standard General had another go, but again there were insufficient funds to meet this small amount. In May, Standard General sent Markuschowitz a letter telling him the policy was in a state of lapse. A few days later, Masail's check for R1 065 arrived to cover the payments for the months of April, May, and June.

Just over a month after his Standard General policy came into force, Markuschowitz put in a dread disease claim. Such an early claim should have galvanized everybody from the claims manager downwards onto full alert.

Markuschowitz maintained he had cancer, and the symptoms had appeared about two weeks earlier. On 14 May, a section of tissue had been removed from his left thigh in the Linksfield Clinic by none other than Dr. Lieberthal, the learner orthopedic surgeon, who was hardly a cancer specialist.

Records from the Clinic showed Markuschowitz had a twenty-minute operation done under local anesthetic. This involved removing what was described as a "firm pale, grey, soft piece of tissue measuring twenty by eleven by four millimeters" that was next to the bone in Markuschowitz's groin. The report from the laboratory of Gritzman and Thatcher was signed by Dr. Marcus Gritzman. The history given was that the 49-year-old patient had a tender lump in the region of the left femur and "the x-ray findings suggest an early lytic lesion".

Like at all the other laboratories that were used by these fraudsters, the people at this one would have had no idea that what was going on behind the scenes was a scam.

A lytic lesion is a growth that breaks down bone. It would be unheard of, a specialist told me, to remove a growth of this kind that was next to the thigh bone under a local anesthetic because the operation would have to be very deep.

However, the lab report stated: "No bony tissue is present, and the tumor appears to be located in the soft tissue". The diagnosis was given as: "Consistent with metastatic, moderately differentiated mucin-secreting adenocarcinoma". The "Comment" was the most disturbing part, as the "exact site of origin" could not be determined. The primary sites which should be considered were the "gastrointestinal tract, lung and possibly prostate". Further tests should be done to establish whether or not the cancer originated in the prostate gland.

If the claim was to be believed, Markuschowitz could have had this killer affliction galloping around his body. The insurance companies did not classify it as a dread disease without good reason.

The x-rays that were referred to in the lab report created another mystery, much like the claims submitted by all the members of the Gang. Dr. Lieberthal said he thought they were done there at the Johannesburg Hospital, but he did not have the film.

At the main x-ray department and at the x-ray section in casualty, there was no record of Bernard Markuschowitz or Bernard Marks having had x-rays done there between 7 May 1993, when he said he first discovered the lump in his leg, and 14 May, when part or all of it was removed. A radiologist told me that doctors who worked at the hospital sometimes had x-rays done for their friends without completing any records. The office equivalent was copying your child's school project on the copier at work.

Having told me that no radiologist's report was done, Wynne contradicted himself by saying Markuschowitz must have the x-rays and, if there was a report on them, it might be in the packet with them.

When I contacted Markuschowitz, the story became more suspicious than ever. He claimed they were destroyed when there was a fire in his office.

Unwilling to accept that unlikely tale, I said, "The Johannesburg Hospital has no record of you having been x-rayed there. How do you explain that?"

"All I know is that I went there one evening by myself and had them done. I have no control over their record keeping."

In my subsequent report to Standard General, I wrote it would be easy for a doctor to send a piece of tissue to a laboratory with his own report, saying that the x-ray findings suggested an early lytic lesion when in fact no x-rays were done. Also, why didn't Markuschowitz have the x-rays at the Linksfield Clinic where the biopsy was done? This was particularly significant in view of the fact that Wynne told me that at the Johannesburg General they often did not provide a radiologist's report. If this was the case, then it would have been even more desirable for Markuschowitz to have been x-rayed at a private hospital rather than at an inefficient provincial one.

Markuschowitz belonged to Consolidated Employers Medical Aid that would no doubt have paid for any x-rays he had at a private hospital, so he had no need to go to a government one. In addition, on 24 September 1993, only four months after his cancer was discovered, Dr. Lieberthal sent Markuschowitz to Dr. Illes and Partners at the same private Clinic to have his back x-rayed because of disk problems.

"Had he had any previous history of cancer?" I asked Wynne.

"Not that he disclosed to me." Why didn't he mention an earlier occasion when he sent tissue from Markuschowitz to the lab, not to either of the ones he claimed he normally used?

I traced a report from the laboratory of Mauff and Partners. It was dated 3 May 1993, just four days before Markuschowitz claimed to have found the lump in his groin. The referring doctor was given as Dr. W. Lieberthal and the patient was named as Mr. B.H. Markuschowitz. "Urgent. Histology? Melanoma" was written on the label on the container in which Dr. Lieberthal sent the specimen.

No information was given as to what part of the body it had come from. The report referred to a "resection of soft tissue vicinity of previously avulsed naevus". This was medical jargon for a piece of soft tissue that had been surgically removed from the vicinity of a place where a mole had previously been torn or broken off. No evidence of cancer was found. Didn't one of the claims from another member of the Gang involve a mole or something similar that had broken off? Was this perhaps a trial run?

I interviewed Markuschowitz in November 1993 at his Design Print offices in the Glenhazel Shopping Centre not very far from where Hugh Lieberthal lived. He was a rotund man with a good head of black hair. My initial impression of him was that he was as slippery as an eel.

"Have you had any follow up treatment?" I asked.

"Yes, I have. I've been to Israel and I've had treatment there."

"What sort of treatment did that involve?"

"They gave me chemo treatment." He looked towards the door as if he was hoping somebody would come in and rescue him from this unwelcome interrogation. The treatment went on for four weeks, he told me, and he was going back there soon for more treatment. He felt more comfortable there because that's where his ex-wife and his children were. Lieberthal had been his doctor since 1980 or1982, he added.

I switched the conversation away from Markuschowitz's Standard General claim, planned to come back to that later if I could keep him talking that long. I had found in my investigations that the more people like him talked, the more they were likely to trip themselves up.

He confirmed he had been in partnership with Hugh in Double Jay Printing, where he had worked briefly, but he had severed his ties with this business two months earlier. He and Hugh had then started Design Printing, the business he was now running.

"Did you apply, or was your name put on a list of people who were part of the Double Jay Group Scheme with Time Life?" I asked.

"Yes," he said, looking concerned. "And I have a policy with Time Life."

He told me he was treated in Israel at the Tel Hashomer Hospital and was scheduled to go back there shortly for further treatment.

"In fact, I'm not even sure that I'm willing to carry on with the chemo." Here was another of the cancer victims talking about abandoning treatment. "I've seen too many people suffer badly afterwards, you know. And the recovery rate is not that great."

He was now being counseled by his rabbi.

Returning to the doctor who had removed the specimen from his leg, I said, "Where does Dr. Lieberthal practice?"

"From home in Victoria Avenue, Sandringham."

"Oh, he runs his GP practice …"

"No, he doesn't run a GP practice, at all. I don't think he runs a big practice. I think he looks after mainly his old friends and family. That's all I know."

It was on the tip of my tongue. I nearly said, "What? He's been working as a GP when he is only supposed to be working under supervision as a hospital registrar?" I just stopped myself in time. In PI-poker, like in the card game, you try not to put your cards on the table until just the right time.

In spite of the fact that Markuschowitz's policy was so new when he claimed and the premiums were not paid from the beginning, Standard General gave him a check for R200 000 at the end of June. These life companies have so much money they can throw it away like this, was what went through my mind. They don't seem to consider that paying dud claims can affect the returns that their loyal and honest clients get on their policies when they mature.

The payment was approved by the Claims Manager Glen Leite after the company took legal advice as to whether or not the policy had lapsed when the claim was lodged. There were no grounds to repudiate it for the late payment because of a technicality in the wording of the policy.

The company was so involved with this aspect that it missed the fraud side of the claim completely. Was Leite perhaps hypnotized by the fact that Masail was one of the principles of a very prestigious brokerage?

When I went back to Markuschowitz's business premises two months later, they were empty. A man in the shop next door told me that Design Print had closed after it went bust. Markuschowitz was believed to have returned to Israel.

He never claimed from Time Life, although the policy had probably lapsed because he never paid the first monthly premium of R357. I assumed that having hit pay dirt with Standard General, he did not want to press his luck any further.

If he was to be believed, he already had cancer when he signed up with Time Life, which showed it had been asking for trouble by granting all the members of the Double Jay Scheme a continuation option with no medical evidence. It was conned well and truly by Masail, who was no doubt helped by people within Time Life.

Dr. Lieberthal allegedly did two procedures to enable his sister-in-law and Markuschowitz to make their insurance claims. Yet the conditions of practice the Medical Council had set for him did not allow him to treat either of them outside the provincial teaching hospitals which formed the circuit that came under the Wits Medical School.

To get his side I asked him, "What are you entitled to do now?"

"I'm busy specializing at the moment and I can do limited private practice, which is a condition of employment at the hospital."

Striking while he had given me this opening, I said, "Since when have you been allowed to do limited private practice?"

"Well, as far as I know, the last correspondence I received from them specifically stated I could do it."

"Yes, but when was that?"

Impatiently he replied, "May I continue, please? That I reckon was about two months ago, two-and-a-half months ago."

He maintained that, from the time restrictions were first imposed upon him, it was never stated anywhere that he could not do private work. "It was, however, in subsequent, um, um, the last letter I received from them that they actually stated it. And, I must say, I, I don't have a private practice anymore."

After his restrictions on prescribing certain scheduled drugs were lifted to allow him to do this in the hospital where he was working, he gave the odd script to members of his family. These were for such things as antibiotics and headache tablets.

"None of the letters I received from the Medical Council said I couldn't do that. I would be very grateful if you could obtain those letters because it specifically did not state that."

Had he been reading the same Medical Council requirements that I saw?

I showed him the Medical Council letter, which gave his conditions of practice as of 27 September 1993. Among other things, it stated: "participation in the scheme for limited private practice for registrars within the hospital set-up will be considered on the recommendation of Professor Erken."

Even that was not going to get him to admit he had done anything wrong.

"But this is not correct," he said. "This is what I'm trying to say to you. At the hospital, I didn't actually need Professor Erken's permission." The Medical Council had never said that. All it required was for Erken to give them a three monthly report on his progress, he maintained.

"He can't report on your progress if it happens outside the hospital without his knowledge," I pointed out.

"No, we're not talking about my medical progress. My personal health was what it was about. That's why they required those reports to show I was working well; that I was not taking drugs, and that I was not receiving drugs from the pharmacy. My academic, um, qualifications and medical progress were not being monitored by them."

"Obviously, that all goes with the job. I mean surely the Medical Council is not interest in your health, per se. They're interested in it as it related to you as a doctor," I added, stressing the obvious.

Stubbornly swimming against the tide, he replied, "No."

"In other words, for the protection of the public?"

"Not at all. They cannot refuse me the right to practice. I was practicing fairly, as I am now."

"I'm not disputing that," I said. "But my question is: Were you allowed to operate at the Linksfield Clinic, for instance, on that person who was insured?"

"Absolutely. I have no doubt in my mind that I was allowed to do that. It's certainly not illegal." His anger was coming to the surface now. "I have not been struck off the roll." He gave me a contemptuous look. "And the allegation you make is that I did this illegally."

In the middle of our verbal wrangle, he suddenly came out with a startling confession that I had never asked him about. Was he really unbelievably bright? It was something nobody had so much as hinted at during my inquiries.

"I applied for the job as a registrar without disclosing that I had had an addiction problem. Professor Erken subsequently found out about it. He called me into his office and I confirmed that I had had a problem. Nevertheless, on my past record of practice, he accepted me for the post."

Wynne continued to deny that the Medical Council had ever set conditions relating to him doing private work.

Chapter 9

Another Doctor Catches It

Dr. Attila Szabo was not content with having just one or two policies like the others. His desire to become an overnight millionaire was such that he signed applications with five different companies for total life cover of R1.2-million and dread disease for the same amount. He took the policies over a six-month period in 1993, with the last application being signed in September of that year.

He was going to make a killing, although life insurance was never designed with this type of killing in mind. By the time he had finished shopping around for policies through his broker Mike Masail, he had committed himself to paying premiums totaling R1 600 a month, a miserly outlay for a jackpot of over a million. His rash of life insurance applications began in April 1993 when he got life and dread disease cover from Standard General, Fedlife, Crusader, Time, and Southern.

Not that he was planning to die, but the only way to get dread disease cover was via a life policy.

Applications normally make dull reading, but his were interesting because they were spiced with a sprinkling of false information. He was aided and abetted by the group's fiction writer Mike Masail. He signed all Szabo's applications as a representative of the Financial Workshop.

The Crusader proposal Szabo signed in July 1993 asked: "If you have applied for Dread Disease benefits please state how much Dread Disease insurance you have with us or any other company?" His answer was "R170 000." He never mentioned the R300 000 Fedlife policy he had taken the previous month. And this must have been in force because he answered "No" to another question which asked if there was any proposal on his life still pending.

In July, when he made his second Standard General application, he had no option other than to mention the first one. He again failed to record the existence of his Fedlife policy and he did not mention his Crusader policy, either.

In his September Southern Life application, the deception continued. He answered "Yes" to the question which asked: "Are you presently negotiating for any other insurance on your life or planning to do this with this or any other insurer?" He amplified this by stating: "31-8-93, Time Life, R100 000." He was then asked if any other insurance had been affected on his life in the last 12 months and he stated: "Stan Gen R130 000 and Crusader, now cancelled." Again he forgot his Fedlife policy, and he left out his other R170 000 Standard General one, as well.

He did not continue with his Crusader policy; I assume because the company's listing on the Johannesburg Stock Exchange was suspended. And towards the end of 1993, it was placed under curatorship by the Financial Services Board amid numerous scandalous allegations.

In April 1993, Szabo took out an Old Mutual income replacement policy to give him a monthly income of R10 000 if he was unable to work. In the application, Szabo gave his salary as R168 000 a year. He stated he obtained his MBBch medical degree in Hungary, and had been studying for seven years in both Hungary and at the Wits Medical School.

Two years before he signed the Old Mutual form, he had been a medical officer at the Hillbrow Hospital and, since 1992, he had been a full-time surgical assistant at the Linksfield Park Clinic, a private hospital as opposed to a provincial one like Hillbrow. There, according to his Standard General application, the good looking, thirty-year-old was helping orthopedic surgeon, Dr. Nainkin.

He was on the threshold of a career as an orthopedic surgeon. As a recent immigrant, the Medical Council had given him a registration which restricted him to working in Gauteng (formerly Transvaal) provincial hospitals until the end of May 1995. Was he working unofficially for Nainkin? Did Nainkin not bother to check the official status of his assistant before he employed him?

When I questioned Szabo about his registration, I started with an innocuous question as a lead in: "When did you start practicing as a doctor in South Africa?"

"In 91, October 91."

"You came from Hungary, did you?"

"Yes."

"What condition did the South African Medical and Dental Council lay down as far as where you could practice and that sort of thing?"

"I've got a limited practice, a limited registration." He had confirmed what I had already found out.

"Limited to what?" I said sharply.

"I can't do private practice by myself." Like Lieberthal, he seemed to be making up his own rules.

"Isn't it correct that you are only allowed to practice in provincial hospitals? I checked with the Medical Council and that's what they told me."

Hesitantly, he replied, "No. What I, what I heard when I was there, they told me that they give appointments with limited registration because some people took up GP practices and they were not allowed to."

Professor Becker, the President of the Council at that time, told me that foreign doctors had to work for a period under supervision at a provincial hospital. "They were not entitled to do private practice at all." If they wanted to get an open registration after they had served their time at a provincial hospital, they had to pass an examination which would put them on a par with doctors who had qualified in South Africa.

It was abundantly clear, just as my conversation with Szabo was in February 1994, that he had no right to be working in Nainkin's private practice while under the restriction Becker talked about. He was also not allowed to operate on Dr. Lieberthal the year before because, although this was done in a provincial hospital, there was no supervision from a senior doctor.

There appeared to be nothing significant in the medical reports done on Szabo at the application stage. He was given a clean bill of health after undergoing various tests, including an ECG. He was a young professional man who could be expected to have a long and healthy life.

The health of Szabo's fellow insurance addicts had a habit of changing drastically for the worst almost overnight, and his turned out to be no exception.

With Masail's knowledge of life insurance, I would have thought he would have advised his clients that life companies were always very suspicious of early claims. If he did pass on this bit of wisdom, Szabo either could not afford to pay the premiums for very long, his greed got the better of him, or there was some other reason I was not aware of. In any event, he started claiming in September 1993. He was supposed to have had a cancerous lymph node removed from his left groin.

The medical reports to support the claim were all completed by Dr. Steven Brower. His connection to the Gang was that he was not only Wynne's friend, but he was also one of Masail's clients. The reports for Standard General, Fedlife, and Southern were dated 6 October 1993. For some unknown reason, Time Life was given a miss.

In them, Brower stated he was not Szabo's usual doctor. He saw Szabo for the first time on 28 September 1993 for what he described as a "routine medical examination". It was then that he discovered an "isolated lymph node" in Szabo's left groin. He removed it the same day in the casualty department of the South Rand provincial hospital. It was sent to the laboratory of Van Drimmelen and Partners where it turned out to be a "non-Hodgkin, malignant lymphoma". This was confirmed by both Doctors Piet Grobler and Don Hamilton. It qualified perfectly as a dread disease according to the cancer definition given by the insurance companies.

In spite of the fact that all the medical forms had the same date on them, Brower was unable to answer one particular question correctly on the Southern form. It asked: "Are you aware of any claim for a similar benefit having been lodged or to be lodged with another company?" He ticked the "No" square. Unlike me as the investigator, the life companies would not have had the benefit of seeing all the forms when they initially considered their claim. They would only have had their own company's form to go on. So, if a doctor stated that he knew of no other claims being lodged, they would have every reason to rely on this information, coming as it did from a member of what many believed to be an honorable profession.

A note made by one of Southern's staff towards the end of October records a conversation the company's doctor Jack van Niftrik had with Brower. Masail had phoned Brower to ask him to examine Szabo for an insurance policy. This made no sense because, by the middle of September 1993, Szabo was already up to his ears in policies. An added factor was that, in the Southern proposal, which was date stamped as having been received at the Johannesburg office on 2 September 1993, Szabo stated he was not contemplating taking any further policies. The insurance medical story became even more improbable after I had spoken to Szabo about it.

"What did you go and see Dr. Brower about?" I asked him.

"For insurance, an insurance medical."

"*Ja*, what company?"

"I don't know."

Raising my voice, I asked, "You don't know?"

"I don't know which one."

"Who sent you there?"

"I went with Mike… Mike… Mike Masail."

I pressed him further. "You go for a medical and you don't know what company it was?"

"I can't remember which company was that."

People did not normally get sent for an insurance medical examination until they had first completed an application. This prompted me to ask, "Had you signed any forms?"

"I probably signed yes."

"But you don't know the company?"

"I can't remember exactly."

According to the Southern Life note, Brower told Van Niftrik that Szabo arrived without a medical form and Masail said he would bring one round later. This was in spite of the fact that these forms were supposed to be signed in the presence of the doctor when the examination took place.

Another Southern note described the claim as "highly suspicious" and that it should be thoroughly investigated. "If there are any irregularities, these should result in the broker being S referenced." S referencing was insurance speak for having a broker blacklisted by all the life companies. This usually only happened to the worst rogues.

The claim forms muddied the water even further. In fact, they also made it decidedly smelly. They were all dated 6 October. On the same day, Szabo signed a Special Power of Attorney authorizing Masail: "To finalize my insurance claim, endorse all checks on my behalf and to enter into any financial transactions with the funds due to me from the aforesaid insurance claim."

Szabo told me that he signed the Power of Attorney in case he was in Hungary when the claims were paid. He denied having borrowed any money from Masail.

Only four claims forms were completed and signed, allegedly by Szabo. They were for Southern, Standard General, Fedlife and even Crusader. Strangely, in the one for Southern, Szabo stated he was making no claim to Old Mutual, Time Life, or in relation to the R130 000 Standard General policy. Was he getting cold feet? He did not disclose his intentions regarding these other two companies to Standard General.

In the Southern claim form, he revealed that when his cancer was discovered he was working at the J.G. Strydom provincial hospital in the Rossmore suburb of Johannesburg and he was also assisting Dr. Nainkin.

Determined not to give another bundle of Standard General's money away, as he had done in the Markuschowitz case, claims manager Leite sent Masail a telex on 20 October which really stirred things up. He informed Masail that, in order for him to assess Szabo's claim properly, his client would have to be examined by cancer expert Professor Werner Bezwoda, the head of the oncology department at Johannesburg General Hospital. He had made a provisional appointment for Szabo for the following day, and needed to know if Szabo would be available before he confirmed the arrangement.

Masail went on the offensive. Laying down the law Masail-style, he maintained there was nothing in the policy document that gave the company the right to demand further medical tests in the event of a claim. If Standard General could not provide a document to substantiate this, his client would "have no option" other than to take legal action in the event of the claim not being met. Masail was, no doubt, relying on the way insurance companies tended to pussyfoot around brokers, particularly the top earners, so as not to offend them in case they stopped putting business their way.

Szabo did not go and see Professor Bezwoda. He decided instead to consult Dr. John Blott, a specialist physician. He saw him at his rooms at the Linksfield Clinic without first telling Leite he was going there, so the company had no chance of giving Dr. Blott any background. Standard General subsequently got Blott's report, which was also sent to Brower. It began: "I saw Dr. Szabo on 2.11.93. He has a 3-4 history of cervical and inguinal lymphadenopathy which he noticed himself". Dr. Blott told me it meant that he had a three to four-month history of swollen lymph glands in his neck and groin. This was very different from the version given by both Brower and Szabo in all the documents they signed for the claims and a far cry from the "isolated lymph node" mentioned by Brower.

When I spoke to Szabo some time after he had seen Blott, I said, "Your lymph gland that you had removed, when did you discover there was a problem with that?"

He was lost for words. There was a long silence. Then he said, "Exactly, I didn't really recognize it. Then I went to go and see Steve Brower."

"What do you mean, you didn't recognize it?" I got in quickly. "You're a doctor, aren't you?"

"Yes. But you can, I mean, it was a node here," he said, pointing to his groin. "And you don't examine yourself every day. So, I don't know."

"Anyway, you went there, and he found this lymph node. What did he tell you about it?"

"He thought that he should cut it out for a biopsy. Then he cut it out a few days later in South Rand." Once again, the members of this dubious claims production were showing what amateurs they were by not co-coordinating their lines.

Deliberately emphasizing each word, I said, "A few days later?"

"I think." For a would-be surgeon, his memory was alarmingly faulty.

"What section of the hospital was it done at?" I shot back at him.

"It was in casualty."

"And did Dr. Brower do it by himself?"

"Yes."

I had earlier been to the South Rand Hospital, which was not far from Brower's surgery. There I asked Hennie Broekman, the Superintendent, if there was any record at the hospital of Szabo having had an operation there on 28 September. He asked somebody to look at the casualty theatre record book and there were two entries for that day. Neither of them was for Szabo. Broekman said that if the operation had taken place at the hospital, it should have been entered even if the operation was on a doctor. Szabo should also have paid for using the hospital facilities.

He said he knew Dr. Brower because he had worked at the South Rand Hospital some years earlier. "It was very strange that he should bring one of his patients to our hospital because Dr. Brower is a major shareholder in the Mulbarton Hospital, which is nearby."

"Did you complete any records there?" I asked Szabo.

"I didn't."

"Did you pay?"

"No."

"You realize you have to pay."

"You see, Steve took me there. He said that we can do it there. I didn't know that I had to pay. If I knew, I probably pay."

Dr. Blott found out that Szabo had a full blood count on 23 November; a few days after Leite had wanted him to see Professor Bezwoda. Dr. Blott told me he had telephoned Brower and told him that this had been irresponsible of him to remove the lymph node without first having this done. Blott had the laboratory tests that were done on the node reviewed by Professor Kum Cooper at Wits University and he was unable to diagnose malignancy.

When Blott saw Szabo, he had already given up his job as a surgical registrar at the J.G. Strydom Hospital and had booked a flight back to Hungry to have treatment with his family near him. "The findings are highly suggestive of leukemia but I thought it was pointless pursuing this further here, as he will be in Hungary in a week's time," Blott decided.

After I had filled Blott in on the case history, he telephoned me to say he had seen Szabo in the corridor of the Linksfield Clinic that day. Szabo told him he had been to Hungary, where he had seen another doctor who did not know what was wrong with him. Blott suggested that Szabo should come to his rooms there and then so that he could take blood for further tests. Szabo declined to do this.

Brower's account of what happened was just as full of holes as the story Szabo had told me. I spoke to him at his surgery in Turffontein and he said, "Okay let me tell you briefly. I've had calls from doctor what's his name, Van Niftrik, and the story is very simple. This person was brought in by, um, his broker for a routine medical." The broker was Masail, who he knew, but he didn't know what company it was for.

"Didn't you have the form with you?" I asked.

"No. What happened was, Masail phoned me and said would I do a medical on him, but he doesn't like the forms used."

That sounded like utter nonsense. Brokers had to use the forms provided by the companies whether they like them or not. He told Masail to bring Szabo in at lunchtime. He knew the medical forms, so if he examined Szabo he could fill in the form later. That was what he did.

"He in fact had multiple lymph nodes," he continued. Now the nodes had suddenly multiplied, so I was waiting to hear how he decided which one had to be removed. "I don't know how familiar you are with medical things but anyway, I said to him, 'Before you go we should remove one of these things, okay?' which we did. I took him to South Rand where they've got a casualty theatre. I just found time to do it. It depends on the procedure. Sometimes I do it in my rooms, sometimes I don't. But when it involves um, in this case the groin, okay, you shouldn't do that in your rooms. Okay? Then we sent that away, and we got that report, which I gather you've got a copy of."

"Yes," I said, congratulating myself on how freely he was answering my questions. I had fully expected him to have clammed up a lot earlier knowing what doctors were like, especially when they were on a sticky wicket.

"That obviously came as quite a shock, I must say." He gave Masail the result, and he instituted things on the insurance side while Brower merely completed the medical certificates. "Then I had numerous calls from, from the various companies."

Dr. Van Niftrik suggested to him that Szabo should go for another opinion. This was done, and he got a letter from Dr. Blott. "I think you've got to understand that I'm a GP, and he's a specialist, (and) that this is certainly not my domain, okay?" The slide was reviewed and Brower "found that really interesting" because firstly one pathologist had the result confirmed by another one and then it was sent it to a third pathologist who disagreed.

"What made you take this lymph node out in such a hurry?" I asked.

"*Ja.* Dr. Blott's letter talks about 'shotty'. Now 'shotty' means small... um small, numerous... small. But this one was, um... was... was may be just bigger than... than others. But this was, this is not an uncommonly, an uncommon thing." He told Szabo he could take it out because he was familiar with surgery.

He was looking at some notes on the desk in front of him and I said, "Is that all the notes you've got, just three lines?"

"*Ja*, that's all I require for this, because I never followed him. I never saw him aft... I saw him okay for that time, sent him away, got the report and, from then, it was left up to him." He had not sent the specimen to the laboratory used by the South Rand Hospital because he had worked at that hospital and he had found the service to be "very below average." Ninety-nine percent of the time doctors used the private laboratories.

I was getting used to conflicting answers in this investigation and Brower maintained the pattern. First, he said he had not recommended that Szabo see a specialist, but his very next sentence was, "He was advised to go and see a specialist, the specialist would then handle the case completely."

"Was the advice given by you for him to go and see a specialist?"

"Mm, no. partly, you know I don't say, I can't say to the guy you have to, you know what I mean."

He was not sure if Szabo had got a copy of the laboratory report, but he gave him the diagnosis over the phone.

I still felt that Dr. Brower had by no means told me everything he knew, so I had one more try to see if I could get the GP to tell all. When I telephoned him and it was evident that things had become too hot for him, he told me he had been advised to tell me that he would only answer any further questions I had with the assistance of the Medical Protection Society, if I put them in writing.

"Do you need medical protection?" I asked.

"No," he said, "But, that's the way I've chosen to go."

The Medical Protection Society is a United Kingdom-based, not-for-profit, mutual organisation that is the world's leading indemnifier of health professionals. It offers legal representation to its members and compensation to patients who have been harmed by their malpractice. According to the Society: "Members commonly seek help with clinical negligence claims, complaints, medical council inquiries, legal and ethical dilemmas, disciplinary procedures, inquests and fatal accident inquiries."

My letter was answered by Graham van der Spuy, one of the directors of MacRobert, De Villiers, Lunnon & Tindall, the Pretoria law firm that acted for the Medical Protection Society. In the high-handed style of his breed, he told me that Brower was not obliged to "reply to interrogatories of the nature of those in your letter under reply".

Other aspects of the conversation I had with Szabo made me wonder how much he had actually learnt at medical school. He had already been back to Hungary when I saw him.

Testing his medical knowledge, I said, "You're a doctor, so can you tell me whether it's good medical practice to take a lymph node out before you've had a full blood count?"

"No, it can happen."

Gruffly, I snapped, "I know it can happen, but is it good medical practice?"

"Sometimes from blood you can't say anything, you can't tell."

"No, but unless you've done the blood count, you won't know, will you?"

Tongue-tied, he claimed ignorance. "You see, I didn't… no we've been… no I don't know."

I asked him to show me his passport. This proved he had left Jan Smuts airport in Johannesburg on 11 November and had returned on 23 November. At least that part of his story was genuine.

"What did you go to Hungary for?" I enquired.

"I wasn't very happy about the first report on my condition. I discussed it with my family and I just wanted to go home. And I went to see doctors there, as well."

"What doctors did you see?" It seemed a simple enough question, but all I got was another long silence. "What are their names?" I demanded.

He saw a Dr. Babay in Budapest where there were reports on his condition. His answers became more suspect when he said these weren't ready when he left Hungary. Our conversation got even more absurd when I tried to find out the name of the hospital where he saw this Dr. Babay. All he would say was that it was a "big, big, hospital."

To add to the ridiculous, this doctor was supposed to have been a friend of his when he was living in Hungary. He discussed Blott's report with this doctor, who showed it to other doctors there. "He's not a specialist in this, he's actually also a surgeon."

As my questioning of Szabo continued, it became clear that, apart from submitting dodgy claims, he had other talents which were also completely toxic as far as the Hippocratic Oath was concerned.

He had not been conducting himself "as becomes a member of an honorable profession" in his dealings with his superiors. Perhaps they did not have this oath in Hungary, or his thinking was that, if some of his colleagues were ignoring it, why should he be nobbled by this outdated brake on progress? He confessed to the kind of morality that was far from ideal for anybody, let alone a surgeon.

Professor Desmond Pantanowitz was head of the Surgery Department at the J.G. Strydom, the provincial hospital where Szabo had been working before he went to Hungary. The Professor informed me that Szabo told him that he had to go to Hungary urgently because his father was desperately ill. He offered to arrange for Szabo to have special leave, but the learner-surgeon went to the staff office and resigned without telling Pantanowitz. The truth was revealed when I grilled Szabo on this.

"How were members of your family when you went to Hungary?" I said. "Were they in good health?"

"Yes," he answered, evidently unaware of how well I had done my homework.

"You were working at the J.G. Strydom at that time, were you?"

"Yes."

"Did you tell anybody there that you had to go to Hungary because your father was seriously ill?"

"Yes, I did."

"Why was that?"

"Because I didn't want to tell them I thought I was sick. Why should I tell them? I thought I might come back to work there. I don't think it's a good idea." He conceded he had resigned without telling his professor. He maintained that Pantanowitz had told him that this was his only option.

This was as good a time as any for me to deal with another one of his work related fabrications. For a change, this one got him into trouble.

"I think you worked at the Boksburg-Benoni Hospital?"

"Yes, I did."

"Why did you leave there?"

"Because I knew a few people, who worked there," he said, conveniently misunderstanding the question. "That's why I came into this country the first time."

"But why did you leave that hospital?"

"Because I didn't get a job there. I've got a job for six months. Then I was on leave. After that I didn't get a job."

It was time to up the tempo of my interrogation once again, so I said, "There was no question of you taking sick leave and being seen at some water polo function in Durban, was there?"

"I discussed this fact with the Superintendent. I was sick and I went to Durban."

"To play water polo?"

"I didn't, *ja*, I played."

The Superintendent had spoken to him about this. After that, he did not get his normal leave, and they deducted money from what he was owed. Putting the boot in, I raised my voice. "You lied to them?" He did not reply, so I went on, "In the same way you lied to Professor Pantanowitz about your father being desperately ill."

"No, you see I… I can't say that."

"How many other things did you lie about, Dr. Szabo, regarding these claims?"

"I didn't lie."

"No. You see it's very strange that yourself; Dr. Lieberthal; Mr. Markuschowitz, a big friend of Hugh Lieberthal; Dr. Lieberthal's brother, and Mrs. Lieberthal, who is Hugh Lieberthal's wife, you people all take out this kind of dread disease insurance. And all of you have medicals which show that you are in perfect health before the insurance is given. Then, within a few months, all of you are making claims and you've all got cancer. And all the operations are done in very unusual circumstances. You go to hospitals, there's no record of the operations, and so on. Some of the people are paid. And nobody seems to be having any proper follow-up treatment, although these are very serious conditions and one wonders what the hell is going on here. It looks as though you people, you, in particular, tried to defraud the insurance companies."

"I didn't."

"You didn't?" I shouted.

"No."

"Okay, we will see what happens. Thank you very much."

Unlike his colleagues, brinkmanship evidently proved too unnerving for the Hungarian. He chickened out, which must have been a great disappointment to Masail. Via his broker, Szabo sent Standard General a hand-written letter stating: "In November, the histology of my lymph node biopsy was received at the request of Dr. Blott. The findings, as you are aware, were non-specific. Dr. Blott suggested a routine work up and in addition viral studies. On 11 November 1993 I departed for Hungary, where further investigations were done. These findings also suggested the possibility of a viral infection. In view of this I therefore withdraw my claim on my dread disease policy until such time that further evidence becomes available."

It was a narrow escape for Fedlife. A check for R300 000 had been made out for Masail to collect at the Johannesburg office. Fortunately for his company, Sieberhagen "smelt a rat" because Masail had recently submitted a cancer claim that was paid. He got hold of the check and, when Masail came to collect it, he told him, "I would like to have peace of mind before I hand it over." And this he never did.

Szabo got nothing from any of the companies. He learnt the hard way that the bigger the gamble, the greater the chances are that you will lose your original stake, in this case the premiums that he paid. This penalty was in no way appropriate for what he had attempted. It remained to be seen whether he would have to contend with the full might of the law.

When it came to which dread disease to choose, the companies had not given Dr. Lieberthal and his fellow cancer sufferers much option for their brand of insurance. According to Time Life's definitions, which I assumed must have been much the same for the other companies; there were eight categories of dread disease. There was the total and irreversible loss of sight of both eyes: Not a pleasant prospect and a bit difficult to organize if they hoped to see again once their claim had been paid. A heart attack would do, but then they would have to prove that a portion of their heart muscle had died because of inadequate blood supply. Coronary heart disease that required heart bypass surgery would also get a claim admitted, but that was far too drastic. A stroke with evidence of permanent neurological damage was another one. But even the best medical brains would find it difficult to lay on that to order. Failure of both kidneys resulting in regular renal dialysis; a major organ transplant of some kind, and total paralysis of both arms and legs were other possibilities that had little appeal.

The eighth one was cancer. Now that was definitely the most viable money-making disease for anybody with a bit of medical ingenuity. All that was required was biopsy evidence of an invasive malignancy, which could be as simple as a lump on the skin. There was no disfiguring operation needed and no unnecessary risk to their health. And if you worked in a hospital, specimens that laboratory reports had already proved to be cancerous would have been readily available to doctors. This presented a golden opportunity for the Gang of Seven and they took it with considerable daring.

By involving several companies, Masail and his collaborators managed to get away with a considerable sum before the word spread through the life insurance industry that cancer had infected too many members of the group for it to be a coincidence. It was especially alarming as they had all taken substantial dread disease cover.

The Gang's haul totaled R1 021 566. It must have been a medical first. How the loot was shared only the members knew. As events would later prove, the Medical Council was not prepared to do its own investigation to establish whether the doctors involved had acted unethically by its standards.

Chapter 10

The Brokerage

The Financial Workshop was a life insurance brokerage company formed by hot shot financial experts who had been with the big life companies. At the time of the crisis in late 1993, the eight directors were, Mike Beder, Stanley Chesed, Norman Isaacs, Hilton Yutar, Willem Loubser, Mike Masail, Trevor Traube, and Hylton Rosen, according to a letterhead of a November 1993 letter sent by Masail.

"Mike Beder was our MD," Loubser told me. "He and Stan Chesed were basically running the organisation. The rest of us were also directors, but we each wrote business independently of each other. The money we earned went into a pool and at the end of the month they would deduct each person's share of the rent, telephones, and whatever, and we would each get a check based on the amount of business we had each brought in. I was responsible for my own business. We didn't share it. Mike (Beder) and Stan were the signatories on the checks."

I asked if he had been there when Mike Masail was there. "Very much so, to my detriment. His office was right next to mine. He was fluent with his mouth, you know, and I could see he was doing extremely well financially. But his business was a closed book, really. I didn't know how he did it because I didn't go round asking everybody what they did with their clients, face to face, and they didn't ask me. I went on holiday and when I came back hell broke loose."

"What do you mean by that?"

"Beder and Chesed came to me and said Mike Masail doesn't work here anymore. He resigned and left the country. Then some clients came in and wanted to murder him."

"Did you know anything about him ripping off old ladies?"

"It came out in the wash at the end of the day."

Loubser was an in-house financial adviser at Absa Bank in Roodepoort when I saw him. Heavily built, with plenty of white hair, he was jovial and easygoing. He came across as the genuine, honest broker. Liberty Life had wanted to sue him because of the money that Masail had got away with as he had signed a surety with Liberty. But each partner had signed for their own business, which had nothing to do with anybody else who worked there, and he was responsible for his own lapses.

"What happened when Liberty got on to you?" I asked.

"I just said to them go fly a kite. I had my own contract with the insurance companies. None of them had a contract with Financial Workshop. We all had contracts in our own names. I went to Liberty, Momentum, Sanlam, and Old Mutual and signed in my personal capacity. Liberty sued Financial Workshop because it lost a lot of money with Masail. And Southern Life lost plenty, plenty. It was a lot of money."

"I heard a story that Masail owed a total of around R800 000," I put to him.

"It was more than that."

Asked what happened about Liberty's case, he said, "We all got together at a meeting and I said they can't sue Financial Workshop because who do they sue? I'm a director but my Liberty contract was personal. So they would have had to sue me personally, which they didn't do because I had done nothing wrong. I didn't steal their money. Mike Masail did. I don't know what happened after that. I just said to Beder they must sort it out. I've got nothing to do with it."

"It fell through then, did it?"

"*Ja*, I think so."

Changing tack I said, "At that time, there were funny goings on with Time Life."

"Yes, Masail was well in there. They also lost a lot of money."

When I saw Beder at the end of December 1993, he agreed to help me with my Masail investigation. He had been speaking to all the companies involved to "try and get to the meat of the problem".

"The thing is, we've got the brother on claims, the wife on claims, and both of those two claims are not claims," he said. "We have the husband on claims and one has been paid, but I'm not convinced he has cancer."

"Yes, but what gave you the idea this wasn't so?" I asked.

"You know, the same doctor, seeing one another and that sort of thing."

"What put you onto this?"

For two months, he had known that there were investigations going on. He had been defending Masail. "I was saying he would never do anything like this. Then, he actually threw his hands up in the air and said, bugger everybody, stuff them all. And I thought, this oke's not defending himself. I'm going to have to look into this a bit deeper now and not just take his word."

That was when he started making inquiries. What rang bells for him was when the claim for W. Lieberthal was mentioned, which was the one he hadn't known about. "It's probably the most crucial in the whole pack. He was in and out of this office twice a week, because he was Michael's greatest friend. He's the common thread seeing as H. is his brother; J.N. is his sister-in-law; he knows this Dr. Brower. Dr. Szabo is claiming. He did Markuschowitz's claim. Now there is a trend for me."

"What has Masail got to say about it?" I asked.

"I let one of my financial experts take him to lunch and say, 'What's going on? Why aren't you defending yourself?' His attitude was stuff everybody. 'I'm not involved.' For me, a clean name is very important. I've been defending this guy for two… You know, I'm going to be implicated just now because I'm taking his side and he's not defending himself'." What he did was to insist that Szabo and Mrs. Janine Lieberthal should have a retest. Those were the only two he knew who had been requested to do this so far.

He knew that Masail paid Mrs. Lieberthal the money he got from her claim in cash. "When there was a question of her having to pay it back, she told him to piss off, she'll pay them R1 000 a month. A hell of a strange attitude.

"So I said to Mike, her retest says there's no case there, no sign of cancer. 'You owe Time Life R150 000'. He just walked out. When he went on holiday, he refused to phone Time Life about this."

He put forward two reasons which he described as "guesses, but good explanations" as to why the claimants in the Gang had their money paid into Masail's trust account. It was because these people were "impecunious" and owed their bank money. "You go and put it in your bank account; the bank isn't going to give it to you. If you run to another account and you get the cash, the bank can do bugger all about it. Your overdraft can be R200 000; the 150 000 that came in the bank wouldn't even see. That is my feeling as to what happened. I know that H. Lieberthal is a man who is insolvent. From the short-term insurance side, I consider him a professional claimant. He's unreliable in that every time he goes to a new insurance company he puts in a claim. I have a very good friend, John Appleton. He's an assessor and investigator on the short-term side and he nailed him."

"What can you tell me about Masail lending Hugh Lieberthal quite a lot of money?" I asked.

"*Ja*, that's only by innuendo that I know. He said to me Hugh still owes him some money. Seemingly this is over years. It comes and goes and it's repaid and re-lent. I keep trying to find out why."

"Did he ever say how much Wynne Lieberthal owed him?"

"There've been times when I believe it's up into hundreds." I presumed he meant hundreds of thousands of rand. All he knew for sure was that Masail bought a Fiat Uno car for Dr. Lieberthal because he could not get finance anywhere. "I don't know whether Wynne's paid him back. I know he insured Wynne to cover the loan he made to him. He might even have insured Hugh for the same reason."

When I mentioned Dr. Brower, he said, "He took a hell of a big policy through Mike. It was big enough for me to question before I knew there was any shit. It was big enough for me to say, what are we doing here?"

"What do you mean?"

"You know I'm not on top of all of them, but if I see a big commission check, I have a look at the policy and I ask about it. It was a retirement annuity. But I didn't like the way it was done. It was most certainly oversold. It was wrongly done. That's when I got onto Mike's case."

Brower's Southern Life application was dated 10 October 1993, when Masail must have known he was in deep trouble. The retirement annuity investment was R6 000 a month over a 25-year period for the 40-year-old doctor. In a Crusader Life Medical Report done on Masail in July 1992, he stated that Brower had been his doctor for the last eight years.

"Michael got paid commission," said Beder. "I understand it was over 50 grand, but he just hasn't got any bloody money, anymore. I worked out there's over R850 000 he has to pay now in commission debts and loans and stuff like that. And then there's Time Life, Fedlife, and so on, claims that he has to repay," He didn't know what was going to come up in the next few months, but he was going to contact all Masail's clients.

Life brokers got paid commission up front for policies they wrote and if a policy lapsed within the first two years they had to repay the commission. This long-standing remuneration system in the life industry resulted in companies losing out now and again when brokers like Masail could not repay what they owed.

In the middle of January 1994, Beder sent a letter to Standard General and various other life companies saying that Masail had been suspended "with immediate effect." He informed them that: "A number of most unfortunate allegations have been made against Mr. Masail and, until he can be cleared of all suspicion, the suspension will remain in force."

In early February, Masail had just come off a respirator after being in hospital for some days. The strain of having to tell lies all the time had evidently taken its toll. Either that or he was just taking temporary refuge in hospital because he seemed to recover quickly enough to enable him to skip the country soon afterwards. This was what he had in mind all along. That was why Masail was able to be so forthcoming when Sieberhagen questioned him about the money he had dishonestly obtained. Telling people he would repay them was his final confidence trick, as he knew he had no intention of sticking around for long.

Who was the mastermind behind the dread disease scam? It was almost certainly Masail because he had a previous experience of how well this could work. In his 1992 Crusader application, he was asked if he had ever claimed under any "accident, sickness or disability insurance policies" and his answer was: "Accidental injury for eye/dread disease for melanoma." In the Medical Report that was done in relation to this application, which was for an investment plan and medical insurance, he stated that, in 1990, he had a malignant melanoma on his left calf which was removed with a "wide excision." In addition, he had a "retinal vein thrombosis" in his left eye in 1988.

Masail had been at the Financial Workshop for two years when the dread disease scandal broke. When he made his own dread disease claim, he was working for Southern Life.

Peter Byers was the general manager of Southern at the time. "I recall the hoo-ha about his supposed cancer or removal of a growth from his leg. I can't recall what we did. I remember the incident and that there were a lot of raised eyebrows. People remember rogues, usually with a touch of admiration," was his wry comment.

Loubser, who was also at Southern, thought Masail's claim was paid. It was something he couldn't have done without the help of another bent doctor.

"Well, that's where he got the idea from for these doctors and the others," I said.

"*Ja*, absolutely. It was a conspiracy and the doctors played with him. It was sick. I've been in the industry now for 34 years and, if you bullshit, it will catch you, there is no doubt."

Financial Workshop was started when the directors broke away from the life companies they were with. Loubser, Chesed, Traube, and Masail had all worked for Southern Life. Beder came from Liberty. Loubser was at the brokerage for about three years when he saw that "things were not going the way they should" and he was not getting anywhere. This prompted him to resign as a director and move on.

After that Traube left, then Isaacs, and then Yutar. Finally, the only two directors still there were Beder and Rosen. According to Loubser, all the Financial Workshop directors had been high flyers writing millions of rand worth of business. Beder drove a Rolls Royce and also had a Porsche.

Most of the companies involved in the scam disappeared. Fedlife was absorbed by Investec Bank and Standard General, Time Life, Southern, and Crusader either went bankrupt or were swallowed up by larger companies.

Keith Howes was Standard General's chief underwriter in 1993. It was his job to vet any early claims over R100 000. For some reason or other, Markuschowitz's R200 000 claim did not come to him. It certainly qualified for his approval before it was paid because the broker Mike Masail was chasing the money on behalf of his client in extremely suspicious circumstances.

Masail dealt with Leite, who authorized the payment. Afterwards, according to Howes, Masail took Leite out to a slap-up lunch with crayfish and the works. One could only speculate what went on behind the scenes.

A real gentleman Leite, who was always immaculately dressed, was shot dead in the driveway of his home a few years later while trying to protect his wife from robbers, so I was never able to find out exactly why he paid the claim, as that was not part of my brief when I did my investigation. In any event, insurance company executives were usually too embarrassed to discuss this sort of thing with me afterwards if my report revealed, as was the case here, that the company had made a very expensive mistake.

The next claim Masail submitted was for a total of R300 000 for the two policies Dr. Szabo had with Standard General. This one Leite did refer to Howes. "What surprised me initially was that the lymph gland was removed from the doctor's groin, not by a surgeon, but by a GP," Howes told me. "Also, it was the second big cancer claim in a week from the same broker. You don't just remove a lymph gland without first doing blood tests to find out what's wrong with it."

He sent a letter to Dr. Brower asking for more information. "I wanted to know what blood tests were done before he decided to do the operation; who assisted him; which theatre was used, and whether it was done under local or general anesthetic." He got the same response as I did: a lawyer's letter telling him that Brower did not have to answer his questions.

This was like setting off a burglar alarm because it was contrary to the traditional understanding between life companies and the medical profession. It was generally accepted that doctors who had treated claimants would give the companies concerned full details. This was especially so as the forms policy holders signed gave the companies concerned their consent to obtain their medical history. In this case, Brower had not only been the original treating doctor, but he had also completed the medical report for the purposes of the claim.

"That's when I got even more suspicious, so I phoned around the market to Fedlife, Time Life, and a few more," Howes went on. "They did not have claims for the same people but others who had taken policies with dread disease cover from the same broker. Szabo had claimed from Fedsure and they were preparing to pay. So I called a meeting of the re-insurers at the offices of Cologne Re-insurers and it was decided to bring in an investigator and then go to the police."

After Standard General received my six hundred page report, it was given to the Attorney General's office in Johannesburg. I also handed a copy to George Ratcliffe, the ethics investigator for the Life Underwriters Association of South Africa (LUASA). This association had the job, among other things, of ensuring that brokers maintained the highest standards.

Ratcliffe was originally from Scotland before he moved to Cheshire, where he was a magistrate and a financial adviser with his own brokerage business. In 1990, at the age of 57, he decided to retire early to a sunnier climate. That brought him and his wife Margaret to Johannesburg.

Public spirited and selfless, he began devoting much of his time to crime fighting. In 1993, he was instrumental in starting one of the first policing community forums in the country at the Roodepoort Police station. He eventually had his own office there and dedicated himself to getting the community and the police to work more closely together. He was elected chairman of the Roodepoort Community Policing Forum, then chairman of the provincial board and, eventually, in 1999, he was elevated to the same position on the national board.

At the same time as he was busy helping the police fight crime, he also had the job at LUASA, which had fifteen hundred members. "Every complaint against a LUASA member came onto my desk," he said with an air of authority. "I would investigate them, and we had some success. I did the same job at the Life Insurance Association in the UK. I was a founder member in 1970, a past president, and I also took over the role of chairman of the ethics committee."

He was a man with impeccable credentials. With his contacts, I expected the police to fast track their inquiries into the insurance claims made by Dr. Lieberthal and his cronies. At that stage, the investigation seemed to have stalled.

By this time, Masail had skipped the country.

I asked Ratcliffe if he had done his own investigation after I had given him my report. "I tried. I also took your report and other bits and pieces to the Senior Prosecutor in Johannesburg who was prepared to proceed. I took two guys from the Commercial Crime Branch to lunch at the social club at the Johannesburg General Hospital. I don't know if they started an investigation but the docket just disappeared."

Even with his police contacts, Ratcliffe could not counter whoever was pulling the strings.

"I was very passionate about this because there was a hell of a lot of money involved," Howes told me. "The investigation was passed from pillar to post by the police and nothing materialized. They told Glen Leite that white collar crime had taken a back seat as they were too busy dealing with violent crime."

Sieberhagen also tried to get some action out of the police. "I got the impression there was nobody competent enough to do it. It started with a major and ended up with a little constable who had hardly started."

Lieberthal had done his Houdini act once again.

LUASA proved to be just as ineffective as the police. Only time would tell whether there would ever be anybody to get Dr. Lieberthal and his crooked colleagues to pay for what they had done.

Chapter 11

The Big Splash

They had been simmering away for years. The Health Professions Council had managed to keep the lid on the complaints through a combination of incompetence and incomprehensible decisions.

Then, in October 2002, the media, always scanning the horizon looking for a big one, yelled out across the airways and their pages, "Thar she blows," much like the old whalers would have done. Splash followed splash like nothing seen before in the annals of the South African medical profession, which had a well-disciplined system in place to prevent just such an occurrence. In the country's media history, it might well have been the most publicity ever given to one man who had no political, or sporting, connections,

Overnight, 47-year-old Dr. Wynne Lieberthal, MB Mch, spinal surgeon of distinction, had become a household name. And so had the two story, 128-bed Rosebank Clinic by association—an association that was not exactly undeserved because subsequent events showed that the management of this hospital knew that Lieberthal could well be exposed long before the media finally took the story by the throat and began shaking the life out of it. Slotted in between office blocks, it was not in a quiet, park-like location that you might have expected for a private hospital. Its convenient location to the wealthy suburbs around it perhaps made up for its lack of tranquility.

Talk Radio 702, with a listenership of 280 000 in the financial and industrial hub of the country around Johannesburg and other parts of South Africa, started it all. Then The Star newspaper, the country's largest selling quality daily, took up the story for its 500 000 readers. For 10 consecutive publishing days or more, the paper splashed it across virtually its entire front page, often with equally large spreads inside. Reports which were just as prominent followed on subsequent occasions. The Star's sister paper, The Saturday Star, also climbed in.

Other publications, like the Afrikaans papers, the daily Die Beeld and Rapport, with its Sunday sales of 300 000, also could not resist a good story. The general interest family magazine, You, with a countrywide, weekly circulation of 235 000 and Noseweek, the expose` monthly, cashed in as well.

The surgeon later complained that he got more coverage in South Africa than 9/11, the Bali bombings, and as much as the US/Iraq war.

Lieberthal had the unenviable distinction of being one of the villains in The Star's Top 100 South African Newsmakers of 2002. He came fourth. Number one was Mark Shuttleworth, the IT billionaire, the first African and the second tourist in space. Just ahead of Lieberthal was another rogue, Hansie Cronje, South Africa's disgraced former cricket captain. He died in a plane crash after being banned for life for match fixing.

Sean Cooper was a brilliant all-round sportsman. He was good at just about every competitive outdoor activity imaginable. This was probably inevitable, as his family had an impressive sporting pedigree. His parents, Ron and Stephanie, and his two older brothers, Justine and Grant, were all outstanding in their chosen sports.

Sean excelled at tennis, cricket, cross-country running and swimming while at Ferndale High School in Randburg where he ultimately took his Senior Certificate examination in 1992. He captained several of the teams. His favorite seemed to be rugby. As a scrumhalf, he got his full colors and twice reached the Craven Week trials. His versatility extended to something other than sport because he was described as having a "most beautiful singing voice." This earned him the principal part in the school's production of Joseph and the Amazing Technicolour Dreamcoat.

After leaving school, he got a diploma in sports marketing and various other aspects of sport. So he knew all about the crippling injuries that sportsmen often receive. That did not deter him from specializing in perhaps the toughest and most dangerous of all the sports he had played. His CV for his achievements in the 15-man game after he left school was something that any player would have been very proud of. He was in the Transvaal Under-21 rugby side for two seasons and represented the Barbarians for a one-off game against New Zealand's Auckland Blues Under-21 team. He also played for the first teams of Pirates, Roodepoort, and DHS Old Boys clubs. His other achievements included being picked for the Johannesburg-based Lions Vodacom side.

In between all his rugby activities, he still had time to excel in other sports. He came third in the Junior Iron Man Triathlon and 102nd in the Duzi, the country's premier river canoe race. He competed in the Midmar Dam mile swim and was fourth in the Capital K, the one kilometer training swim for the Midmar mile.

His father was managing director of the Intercontinental Tobacco Company, one of the marketing arms of Rothmans International. He naturally followed his dad into the cigarette industry and became a manager with Peter Stuyvesant. Then in 2001, he took up a position in sales in Johannesburg at Leaf Wireless, which specialized in Windows-based cell phones for large corporate clients.

Sport, but no doubt mainly his rugby, took a dreadful toll on Cooper's body. Finger fractures; shoulder dislocations; concussion; a skull fracture; and, finally, severe back pain, were what he had to endure for the love of the game.

Things finally came to a head in August 2002. His back was giving him so much trouble that he consulted Dr. Lieberthal, the eminent spinal surgeon at his rooms in Rosebank. Lieberthal had come highly recommended. He was admitted as an emergency to the Rosebank Clinic the following day for an operation.

Lieberthal inserted screws in his lower back to fuse the vertebrae, but when Cooper came round, his pain was more intense than ever. It was five days later that Lieberthal confessed that the x-rays showed he had left part of a scalpel in Cooper's back. "I asked him what damage it can do, and he said, "None", Cooper noted in his diary. He was discharged from hospital "over the telephone" the following day, even though he had not recovered.

The sequence of events that occurred during his treatment were vividly described in the diary of pain and anguish that Cooper managed to keep, despite all that he was going through. He had evidently kept it as some kind of insurance after hearing uncomplimentary hospital gossip about Lieberthal.

On Day 7, he was in such pain at home he had difficulty in walking. His calls to Lieberthal were not returned. Three days later, he was taken to Lieberthal's rooms, where the doctor readmitted him and put him back on Pethidine.

Another operation was performed to sew up a hole in the sheath surrounding his spinal cord that was oozing fluid. Lieberthal also claimed to have freed nerves at two levels of Cooper's spine.

"Tells me everything is 100%," the diary recorded on Day 12, even though Cooper still had that razor sharp piece of metal in his back.

On Day 19, fluid was leaking out of his spine once again "all over the bed".

Two days later, he changed to Dr. Brad Hoffman after his mother had "fired" Lieberthal. His new doctor was concerned that the fluid leak, which was causing nausea and headaches, could lead to meningitis. He booked him for surgery the following day.

Peter Cotterell, whose brother was a doctor, was the manager of the Rosebank Clinic. He remembered Cooper because he was worried about the "piece of metal" in his back. Cotterell had become a hospital manager with Netcare, the largest private hospital group in the country, after being managing director of an engineering company for 23 years. His job was to try and keep the peace between the staff and the doctors, and to make sure everything ran smoothly. "I had never been so stressed in my life as I was during my five years managing hospitals," he told me.

When he moved to the Rosebank Clinic in 2002 from Milpark Hospital, it took him about three weeks to find out there was a "nightmare there, and his name was Wynne Lieberthal".

"Some doctors were not very happy with what was going on. On the other hand, there were other orthopedic surgeons, who had been there a long time who, you know, were fine with him. So I was wondering what was going on here?"

One weekend, Cooper asked him if he could get hold of Lieberthal because he wanted to see him. Lieberthal had gone away, so although he tried, he could not get in touch with him. "I had to tell Cooper, 'There's nothing I can do. Doctors are independent people who do whatever they like'. Cooper was absolutely livid. He was then seen by Brad Hoffmann, a neurosurgeon, who was the next guy on call. This upset Lieberthal a lot. He inferred that we had deliberately called in another surgeon."

Five years after Hoffmann first saw Cooper, I asked him about Lieberthal. Like most doctors I encountered, he was reluctant to speak to me. "He seemed to lead a charmed life," he said. "I don't know why, especially as this man is potentially dangerous. The only way I could help was by helping his patients who were in trouble."

While he was in hospital, Cooper had a visit from his cousin Regan Thaw, who came to see how he was getting on. "It was the look of abject pain on Sean's face that struck me as I walked over to his bed," Thaw recalled. "Through clenched teeth and a semblance of a smile, he greeted me, shook my hand, before sinking back in anguish. Without even speaking to Sean, I knew something was seriously wrong."

In his angry state of mind, Thaw was just the person Cooper wanted to see. And, when he disclosed to Thaw what Lieberthal had done, it did not take long before the airwaves were ablaze with inflammatory talk that was to send Lieberthal scurrying for legal advice.

You see, Thaw just happened to be a reporter for the Eyewitness News section of Talk Radio 702. Everybody gets sick from time to time so a doctor's muck-up of this magnitude was bound to interest all his listeners.

"Having witnessed the pain Sean was in, I couldn't ignore the issue. Neither could I ignore an x-ray he showed me where a piece of a scalpel blade was clearly visible, as was its proximity to his spinal cord. I jumped at the story, bracing myself for a long, possibly treacherous and difficult investigation. Imagine my surprise and shock when, after airing the first story, 702 Eyewitness News phone line screeched to life. A Pandora's box had been opened."

Katy Katopodis, Thaw's News Editor, was to say later, "We were confident that we had a good strong story on our hands. So we ran it thinking it would be a once-off, and that we had exposed a doctor for one bad operation. Little did we know?"

Thaw, too, could not have realized then just how big the story would turn out to be. They seldom come bigger with more human interest than this one.

When it was broadcast on 702's news bulletins, the station had a deluge of callers complaining about the same doctor. They had all suffered from a variety of botched back operations. It looked as though the shooting star of the '92 orthopedic class was about to come plummeting to earth even more rapidly than his rise to the prize-filled stratosphere he had once been used to.

Fearing legal reprisals, the station initially did not mention Lieberthal's name. The Star newspaper had no such qualms. Its story on the same day that 702 broke the news was headlined: "Patient to sue surgeon, who left a scalpel in his back."

In the report by Nalisha Kalideen, Cooper was quoted as saying: "You can imagine how shocked I was. I said, 'This thing can move and will sever all my nerves'. He assured me that it would never move. The nurses told me about all the other patients that this man has left paralyzed. Some have had to come back for 11 operations and others are in such a bad way that there is nothing left to operate on."

He was planning to sue the doctor for malpractice and he knew of 57 pending cases against Lieberthal, the paper claimed. It put Cooper's fury in his own words: "I can't describe the anger I feel. This guy drives two Porsches and has three houses. He even owns the company that puts the screws into your back and he doesn't think twice about sending someone to hospital for the screws—whether or not they need them."

After Thaw's first news broadcast, there were follow-up reports. The afternoon bulletin disclosed that the "Rosebank Clinic has distanced itself from a series of damning allegations against one of the doctors practicing at the Clinic. It is now referring all queries to the operating doctor. They say it's a private matter between the doctor and the patient."

At that time, John Robbie, the former rugby international turned broadcaster, was a 702 presenter. Robbie, capped nine times for Ireland at scrumhalf, was sent to join the 1980 British Lions tour of South Africa after a spate of injuries to those originally chosen. That was his introduction to the country where he eventually settled.

On his Afternoon Drive Show, Robbie could not resist taking the mickey out of the doctor without naming him. "I'm glad he wasn't a brain surgeon, hey. Leaving a bit of scalpel in your back is alright, its fine. Imagine if he left it in your brain, it might give your character a bit more steel, hey." Inviting a writ for libel, he proclaimed, "The way these people have spoken, this is Doctor Death. And if that is the case, and I say if, then how can the guy continue to practice if he's incompetent; if he's dangerous? Now, it might be all nonsense, but some of the allegations that came through were that the medical profession looks after its own. It doesn't matter how incompetent you are, you know, as long as you don't actually break the law, then you are going to be okay."

Three days later, presenter Gareth Cliff interviewed Thaw, who 702 appeared to be promoting as their reporter of the month, if not the year. "To tell us more about the story, the man who broke it, Regan Thaw. The doctors are going to try and remove that piece of scalpel blade today from his back. God knows, that's a difficult place to operate."

"It is an incredibly sensitive and precarious place to operate," Thaw replied. "I was speaking to doctors last Friday, and they said it is a bit of a catch-22 situation cos they might not be able to take it out. The way they have to try and cut it out they might sever the nerves themselves. But they can't leave it in there because it's going to cut the nerves, anyway. We are just holding thumbs that they will be able to remove it."

Cranking up the sensationalism, Cliff went on, "There is enormous outrage, Regan, about this doctor. It seems he has a record. Tell us about this."

"Well, this allegedly goes back as far as January this year. Since we broke the story last week, the newsroom has been inundated with calls from people who claimed they had been paralyzed or been left semi-paralyzed by this Rosebank doc. Yesterday, I compiled a list of the people that phoned and I counted 18, and that's just skimming the surface. It's quite a horror story, going in for a back operation, and you wake up the next morning and you can't walk."

Although Cooper now had a new surgeon, there seemed to be no rush to remove the razor sharp piece of metal that was sitting so close to his spinal cord. Hoffmann's initial operation was to close the hole in Cooper's spinal sack. Eight days later, he went home "feeling a lot better and positive that things are coming right," still with the threat of paralysis looming over him from that blade.

His new outlook was soon shattered. Six days later, he was taken back to hospital by ambulance and given morphine this time. On the fiftieth day of his ordeal, he got the news that he must have been dreading most of all. X-rays showed that the piece of scalpel was moving. "Hoffmann wants to operate," he recorded in his diary. "Am bit scared. Hope that all goes well."

Despite The Star having mentioned Lieberthal's name in its first story on the Friday it referred to him merely as "the doctor, whose name is known to The Star", in its report the following Monday. The reason for this about face was that Lieberthal's attorney, Graeme Krawitz, had threatened to apply for court interdicts against both The Star and 702 to stop them defaming his client unless they retracted the statements that had been made about him. All the derogatory allegations, he claimed, were untrue.

Chapter 12

Media Frenzy

As if to entice the raging bull to come at them, if Lieberthal dared, 702 pulled out a bright red cape in the form of an hour-long discussion. It was between presenter Noeleen Maholwana-Sangqu, who later had her own South African Broadcasting Corporation's "Oprah Winfrey"-type television show, News Editor Katy Katopodis, and listeners.

"The top story in 702 Eyewitness News at this hour," Noeleen began. "A top Rosebank doctor has filed an urgent court interdict to prevent 702 from broadcasting any further allegations of gross negligence against him. Dr. Wynne Lieberthal has gone to the High Court to prevent us talking about him, and I brought Katy in because the story is getting more bizarre by the minute. And the question we want to ask this morning is: should a doctor, who has one complaint, two complaints, or whatever against him, should he not be suspended immediately? I'm going to speak to Katy to get the sequence of events as to what happened. I'd like your reaction to this as well."

Katy revealed that since 702 began running the story on Friday morning, they had been inundated with calls. "Now I have been in the 702 news room for six years, and I don't remember another time when the calls just went on and on and on. They went on the whole day. At that stage, we had not mentioned the doctor's name."

"Absolutely not, until this morning," Noeleen confirmed, "but each and every call that came into the newsroom was saying it is this doctor. Had these people gone to the Health Professions Council to lay complaints?" Noeleen asked.

"Some of them had, some of them hadn't. Some of them wanted us to fight on their behalf, which we said we couldn't. The Health Professions Council confirmed they are currently investigating at least 16 cases of negligence against Dr. Wynne Lieberthal. Nomzamo Khumalo of our news team spoke to him on Friday about the blade in Sean Cooper's back. He didn't want his voice recorded, but he said, 'Yes, I admit that happens, but there is nothing sinister about it. These things happen'." With a note of shock in her voice, Noeleen said, "Oh no, they don't. Oh no, they shouldn't. I go to a doctor. I don't want anything left in my body."

"We went ahead with our stories on the doctor and did not name him until this morning," said Katy. "His lawyers threatened legal action unless we retracted. We refused. It is not something we would do because we stand by our story. They are going to the Johannesburg High Court at 10 o'clock. They want 702 Talk radio to stop talking about this and they want you, Noeleen, not to have a talk show on this."

"Linda, good morning."

"I want to thank you for bringing this to the public's notice. I think it is absolutely appalling that this man is allowed to practice. He should be suspended forever. I don't understand how he can go to court. If he was in America, he would be sued out of everything by every patient. I think it is just sad that South Africans take this with a smile and go on their merry way and have a number of operations afterwards."

Passing the credit to where it belonged, Noeleen replied, "Well, thank Regan Thaw and Katy Katopodis, because they are the ones who brought the story to the fore and 702 listeners who actually called in."

"John Robbie was speaking about doctors just last week on Wednesday, just before the story broke," Noeleen told Linda, "and he was talking about the very same issue: doctors acting with impunity and getting away with it."

Going to the next listener, Noeleen said, "Let us speak to Dee. She supports the Doctor. Good morning, Dee."

"I really think you chaps have crucified him. I think you must allow the official people to take it in hand as they have already. I support him. I think he must take you to court."

"But should we allow it to happen, Dee, because, until the public says enough is enough, these doctors will continue to act with impunity?"

"Well, if he is negligent, if there is malpractice, it has to go through the proper channels. You can't try him on radio, which is exactly what you have done."

"I think there is a responsibility from the media to bring things to the public eye. Louis, good morning."

"I am sitting here fuming at your last caller; first of all because, until it is one of her loved one's lying on their backs after this butcher has taken his hands all over her, then she will have a different story. I think this oke shouldn't be suspended; he should be kicked completely off the roll."

Sounding a belated note of warning, Noeleen said, "Louis, let's be careful here. It depends on whether he has been found guilty of malpractice." Her words were wasted on this listener, who upped the tempo of his attack on the doctor.

"You know, Noeleen, my fiancé is lying on her back today, listening to you on the radio. She is one of Wynne Lieberthal's patients, okay? She is 23 years old. She has had eight operations, okay? From tightening of screws to cleaning the wound under general anesthetic; eight times since February of this year. I have gone to my lawyers, who are dealing with it."

People were queuing up to be able to air their stories of medical incompetence. They clearly felt comfortable with the station's policy of allowing callers partial anonymity by only having to give their first names.

"We have got Sam on the line who is an orthopedic surgeon," Noeleen announced. "He wants to give us some balance. That is what he says."

Here was somebody daring enough to break that doctor's code of silence. But listeners must have wondered: was he going to go as far as giving away some of the long held secrets of his profession?

"I am an orthopedic surgeon. In my experience, considering the number of doctors that are there that treat patients every day; the numbers that go sour are a very small fraction indeed."

Asking him to be more precise, Noeleen countered "What is a small fraction, Sam?"

"I don't know. I can't give you the figures. This we can obtain from the Health Professions Council." Most doctors work privately, he explained, and if they are suspended pending an inquiry, they would not earn anything while the process was going on. Then if the doctor wins, who would pay him? It was for this reason that those who had to judge these cases "would like to be as fair as possible". He was not speaking on behalf of the doctor being discussed, as he didn't even know him.

"Do you have a complaint against you?" Noeleen asked.

He said he had been a surgeon for 13 years and she would have known about it if he had. Like a good lawyer, Noeleen was not going to accept evasive answers. "The answer is 'Yes or no', Sam. Do you have any complaints against you?"

"No, Noeleen, no."

"Do you think Sam, as someone else called in and said that doctors unfortunately protect each other, even if they know within the profession that X doctor is not kosher, you still protect each other?"

"No, Noeleen. They usually will not protect misconduct. Most people are upright, and you know yourself, you know of a lot of doctors that are upright. They will definitely stand up and say, look this is wrong, this is not how it should be done."

Cleverly Noeleen boxed him in and he was forced to admit what many people had been saying. "But I wonder Sam, if you knew this particular doctor, would you go to court and say, 'Yes, he has botched up? I saw someone who had gone to him'. Would you do that?"

"If I was called upon."

"But you wouldn't do it voluntarily, even if you knew?"

"No, if I was called upon, I definitely would stand up if there was misconduct."

"But you wouldn't do it voluntarily?"

"No, Noeleen, a whole lot of things come into that. There is a Health Professions Council and better qualified colleagues are there to do that." He had just verified the existence of the medical profession's unwritten law: see no evil, hear no evil, and speak no evil about a colleague. It was much like the Omerta, the Sicilian Mafia's vow of silence.

"Ah, somebody else, not me, Sam. Thank you very much. You have raised a very interesting point."

Listeners, having declared open season on medics in general, were blazing away with every sickening detail that came to mind, although Lieberthal was the only one named.

"Johanna, sorry to have kept you waiting," Noeleen continued.

She was another patient who had a terrible time after Lieberthal operated on her back in 1998. She went to another doctor and, when Noeleen asked what he had to say about her original surgery, she replied, "He just shook his head. He couldn't believe it and neither could the Professor who was head of Baragwanath. He was a bone doctor who has also left the country for Australia."

"Have you made an official complaint?" Noeleen asked.

"No, because I was in no condition to. My daughter did write several times to the Rosebank Clinic and ask for my papers from Dr. Lieberthal's rooms. We got nothing. They had been lost."

There was a general discussion, and then the news was read about Lieberthal's court action to stop the radio station maligning him, and Thaw announced that 702 would defend the action.

This didn't stop Noeleen. "We are not talking about him specifically, in this case. I'm asking a general question about doctors. When should a doctor be suspended?" Her efforts to keep off the subject of Lieberthal proved fruitless as the very next caller spoke about him without mentioning his name, and Noeleen herself went back to discussing him almost immediately.

This time, she had Ariel taking the surgeon's side. "My first point is you are questioning one of the legal fundamentals and that is the concept of 'innocent until proven guilty'. It's a dangerous game you are playing. You say it's playing with people's lives, but the truth is what you are doing on 702 is playing with this doctor's life. What you are saying, whether it's true or whether it isn't, is going to affect his life fundamentally. The whole reason why that law of 'innocent until proven guilty' exists is to protect people from allegations that are unfounded."

Defending the station's approach, Noeleen replied, "The fact of the matter is that we have 16 cases against a particular doctor. Four of those have in fact been thrown out because there was no evidence, but the remaining 12 are still being investigated."

"A lot of these doctors, especially some of the specialists, have thousands of cases, so 12 cases out of thousands is quite a small percentage."

Suspecting that the caller might be in the "club" Noeleen asked, "Are you a doctor, Ariel?"

"No, I'm not. My second point is this: I'm sure if you do your homework and go and speak to the Health Professions Council of South Africa, you'll find that the majority of cases brought against doctors are thrown out." He said he did not have any statistics on this, but as medicine was not an exact science "everybody who goes into surgery knows that things could go very, very, very wrong".

Giving every indication that, if the caller was not a doctor, then he must have been in the medical profession in some other role, Ariel said, "You have speculated again that it was, in fact, the fragment of scalpel causing the pain in this particular patient. You haven't established that as evidence yet."

"It had to be removed," Noeleen retorted. "He went to another doctor and went into surgery yesterday to have it removed."

The conversation became heated when Ariel said that no doctor could guarantee that an instrument wouldn't break or that an implant was going to stay there and not be rejected.

That really got Noeleen going. She became agitated. "No, no, if I need a heart transplant that is the chance I'm taking. It could happen that my body rejects it. But then I don't want a piece of scalpel left above the heart that has been transplanted." She believed that, while a doctor might not be able to guarantee that nothing would go wrong, he "can guarantee that he won't leave a swab; a pair of scissors; a piece of scalpel or anything in my body".

Anne, another caller, switched the conversation to a more general one. "We have patients" rights, Noeleen, but when you go in for an operation you sign to say you do not hold the hospital or the professionals guilty if anything goes wrong, okay. There's no responsibility, you waive that. I don't think you can have one body acting for patients and doctors. We should lobby to have our own body and we should have doctors disclosing their professional history which is the only thing we can base our decision on."

"Absolutely, Anne, I agree with you completely. If a doctor was to disclose to me that he is being investigated for x, y or z, then I'm in a position to say: I don't want you to operate on me. I would rather have somebody else."

"Lynne, good morning."

"I feel we should get a few opinions. I was told I would be crippled if I didn't have a back operation. I went for a second opinion and I still wasn't happy. The third doctor I saw was amazing. He just told me to buy a decent mattress, to drink some Voltaren tablets, and that was in 1992. And my back is fine, so I'm very grateful. I go for other opinions because I had an aunt who was told she had breast cancer 35 years ago. Her first two opinions would have resulted in her losing a breast. So, she went for a third one and she has both breasts left today. That's why I think we should shop around and realize that doctors are in this for the money, too."

Ivan came on with a new angle. "Noeleen, I was the prosecutor in the inquest court for a couple of years in Johannesburg. That's the court that investigates unnatural death, and we had a professor of anesthetics who sat there as an assessor, the expert to give the magistrate advice on the medical procedures. Then, we had a guy one day who had died during an operation. It seemed to me, and it seemed to the court, that the doctor, who had administered the anesthetic, had been completely negligent. I was puzzled. After the case, I went to the professor and asked him how it was possible that this man had not been investigated and found guilty by the Medical Council. He said to me, 'You will seldom get doctors being found guilty because the people who investigate them are their fellow doctors and they will not put the finger on each other'. So, that was a professor of anesthetics from Wits University who said that to me."

"That they rally around each other, that they support each other," said Noeleen.

Ivan brought up the way the law is geared to favor doctors. "Noeleen, you know we've got a very strange situation with these professional bodies, especially doctors and lawyers. They investigate themselves. They have this most peculiar privilege in legislation that they make the rules for their profession and if one of their members does something wrong, they investigate it themselves. If you are a plumber, a mechanic or some other ordinary person, even a teacher, you get investigated by the courts, or a general commission of inquiry, or something like that. But with lawyers and doctors, they investigate themselves. I think that is one of the reasons why the investigation takes years and the conclusion is, nine times out of ten, that the person is not responsible. I feel this is quite wrong."

Noeleen concluded the discussion by saying, "It becomes a numbers game. But it doesn't happen with all doctors. We have to put this into context and realize it certainly is not all doctors. I still do not know from 702-landers what you really think, but thank you very much."

Some of the early reports in The Star slashed Lieberthal's already tattered reputation far deeper than any scalpel that he had ever used. The media onslaught was so savage that Lieberthal was put in a mental position similar to many of his patients. Will I ever be able to recover from this, he must have thought.

In "Doctor 'stuffed-up' nature buffs, too," The Star repeated the details of Lieberthal's 1989 fake wild life photograph. This came a day after Maholwana-Sangqu's broadcast. A 'Surgery Scandal' broke the next day. Headlined 'Doctor ruined my life–gran', it took up almost the entire front page of the paper, while Lieberthal and his legal team were desperately trying to get a court to put a stop to all this adverse publicity.

The story was about how 77-year-old Elizabeth Potts got a "life sentence of pain" while her surgeon was only given a suspended sentenced by the

Health Professions Council.

Lieberthal operated on her back in 1997. Four years later, the Medical Council found him guilty of failing to send her for an x-ray or MRI scan to determine whether the extensive operation was necessary. His sentence was effectively a tap on the wrist. He was suspended from the register for three months, but this was set aside for two years, provided he was not found guilty of another offence during that time. A suspended sentence was quite meaningless, yet it was one of the Medical Council's favorite rulings.

Patting itself on the back for a job well done, it piously announced: "The penalty was appropriate in relation to the seriousness of the offence."

Potts, who was living in Cape Town with her daughter at that stage, told The Star the penalty was an "absolute farce." She had been living in pain for the last five years and was forced to take painkillers every night so that she could get some sleep, after Lieberthal had "completely messed up" her lower back.

She described how she was referred to Lieberthal after having niggling pain in her lower back for years. All he did before deciding to operate was to test her reflexes. Everything was done in such a rush that when she arrived at the Rosebank Clinic on a Monday night in preparation for the operation the following day, no bed had been booked for her. A special arrangement had to be made for her to have a bed in the High Care section.

After the operation, Lieberthal told her he had found "something unexpected." This turned out to be the five vertebrae that Lieberthal fused without telling her. She only discovered this when she was admitted to the Olivedale Clinic shortly after being discharged from the Rosebank Clinic.

She had to go back into hospital because tests showed that she contracted meningitis after Lieberthal had left a hole in the sheath that holds fluid around the spinal cord. "For seven or eight days, I was away with the fairies and the doctors said I wouldn't make it, but I did," Potts told the paper.

Further back surgery at the Olivedale Clinic followed because some of the fusions had not taken. The following year, screws Lieberthal put in had to be removed. This resulted in her back becoming so bent that she was in danger of becoming a paraplegic. To correct this, she had undergone a 13-hour operation at the Chris Barnard Memorial Hospital in Cape Town a few months before Lieberthal's incompetence was exposed in the media.

"I'm wired up from top to bottom and it has cost about R200 000," Potts said.

With the report was a huge color picture of her standing with a crutch in one hand.

Under the front-page headline, "My Ordeal", The Star introduced Debbie Janssens' catalogue of agony under Lieberthal's care. Inside, the paper devoted an entire page to the diary she kept of her treatment. She had three back operations after her spine was crushed in an ice-skating accident in December

2000.

She stated that, after she had previously had a problem taking opiates due to their addictive nature, she went to Lieberthal because he had operated on her husband a few weeks earlier. She had a spinal fusion and was discharged from the Rosebank Clinic on Christmas Eve.

For the next nine months, she was still having back pain, but she was assured by Lieberthal that this was not due to any complications arising from the operation.

This was another patient like Cooper, who still managed to keep a diary, despite her harrowing treatment. Here is what happened after her initial operation, with quotations from her diary.

Early in October, she was back in the Rosebank Clinic because she was in such agony. Lieberthal fused vertebrae at two levels because he claimed one of the rods had broken.

When she came round after surgery, she could not feel her legs. "No one in ICU tells me what he's done. I think I am paralyzed."

He never came to see her again until she was discharged three days later.

The pain in her one leg is so excruciating that, after resting at home for two days, she arranges with Lieberthal's secretary to be readmitted. His inexplicable behavior continues. "He doesn't come to see me and the following day, he didn't even know I was there," she went on.

Then he tells her he doesn't believe her pain could be caused by the screws pressing on her nerves. A myelogram shows how wrong he is.

Saturday, October 20: "Dr. Lieberthal has given me his word that he will come and see me, but he leaves the hospital without stopping by. The nurses phone him and he says there's no way he'll come and see me before Monday. My husband has me discharged. The following day, I had to be taken to the Sandton Clinic casualty department for a morphine injection because the pain was so intense. For the next couple of months, I lived with the pain by getting injections at this hospital and from my GP. I then consulted a neurologist at Rosebank Clinic who put me on medication mostly used by epileptics."

The following week, after two days in the Rosebank Clinic being treated by the neurologist, she is discharged because he can't do anything more for her.

Thursday, February 14: "I see Dr. Lieberthal and he gives me more morphine. I have to inject myself with it."

Tuesday, February 19: "I am booked back into Rosebank Clinic. Both my mother and my husband phone Dr. Lieberthal and beg him not to give me any more morphine. I am now so addicted that I become angry if I don't get my injection on time. Two days later Lieberthal cuts my morphine dose from 15mg every four hours to 10 mg every eight. Because I've had a convulsion before, after going off morphine too quickly, I fight to get the dosage dropped more slowly. He changes it again."

Friday, February 22: "I am sent home with quite a substantial amount of morphine to inject myself. Am told to wean myself off it. I can't stick to the programme, so Dr. Lieberthal gives me more and tells me to do it properly this time. I do. I am still experiencing a lot of pain, and go to four other specialists, but I am constantly referred back to Dr. Lieberthal. I am very angry that no one will help."

On a visit to her parents' home at the seaside holiday town of Knysna, she has a convulsion. She is rushed to a doctor who tells her it is caused by the morphine. She is put on anti-epileptic medication for two weeks to prevent it from happening again. "The side effects are horrendous and my holiday turns out to be a nightmare."

Wednesday, April 17: She is admitted to Rosebank Clinic again to be operated on the next day. Lieberthal says he will perform a decompression at two levels and remove a lump of bone without doing any fusions. "After the operation, he tells me the screws were so loose he had to take them all out and implant new ones. The cost is astonishing. He says he also released nerves from the L4 and L5 region–the ones he initially said were not trapped. I'm getting lots of morphine."

Friday, April 19: "The head sister of Rosebank Clinic phones about the amount of morphine Dr. Lieberthal is giving me. He is confronted by a panel of the hospital managers and the pharmacy manager. He explains why he is giving me so much–20 mg every four hours. My x-rays do not look good."

Sunday, April 21: "Dr. Lieberthal says I will be in hospital for another three or four days. We start weaning me off morphine."

For the next four days, Lieberthal never came to see how she was getting on

Friday, April 26: "I'm finally discharged from hospital with 17 ampoules of morphine to take home. When I get home, I get a call from Dr. Lieberthal. Someone at the pharmacy has phoned the HPCSA and informed them that he's prescribing morphine to me again. He wants me to return it to him so he can administer it to me. My husband tells him 'No'. Dr. Lieberthal calls me back and demands very angrily that I bring the morphine back. I tell him I can't because I am unable to drive after my operation. He screams that I am an arrogant bitch who will ruin his career. I cry and cry. My husband phones to confront him, but he won't take any calls from us. I wean myself off the morphine, but the withdrawals from all the different medications give me a rapid pulse, headaches, vomiting, mood swings, terrible cramps, and sweats. I feel like I'm dying."

Monday, May 6: "I phone Dr. Lieberthal's rooms. I want to get my file and see another doctor. When I got home from the hospital I discovered on my x-rays that he'd removed the screws at L4 and L5 without telling me. Now I've had the screws removed from the weakest point in my back. My GP tells me I've lost 80% of my lumbar spine muscle and I need a lot of rehabilitation. Because Dr. Lieberthal has just had his broken arm operated on and he has gone on holiday overseas, I can't get my file. A woman who works for him says his lawyer has it. I phone the lawyer constantly, but given the runaround."

Her roller coaster ride with Lieberthal had now been going on for nearly two years, and it was not yet over. On May 7, she decided to report Dr. Lieberthal to the Medical Council. "It was the most nerve-racking decision I have ever made.

"When my complaint to the HPCSA is received by Dr. Lieberthal, I receive threatening letters from his legal representative, Advocate David Goldblum. They threaten me with both a civil and crimen injuria lawsuit."

The way the Medical Council works is that it passes a complaint on to the doctor concerned for his comments. But if he then abuses the system by terrorizing the complainant with legal threats, the Council should take punitive action to stamp out this kind of thing. In this case, the Council apparently did absolutely nothing. And this was not the only time that Lieberthal tried to put the wind-up with somebody who had complained about him to the Council.

"I refused to back off," this courageous woman continued. "I laid a second charge of harassment against Dr. Lieberthal with the HPCSA. I gave them copies of all the lawyer's letters and my responses. Since that time I have not heard from the HPCSA."

"I have finally found a doctor to help me," Janssens continued. "Not a specialist, but a wonderful GP. She has worked tirelessly to help me through a rehabilitation program. She is the reason I am here today and not dead from an overdose of opiate. I am grateful there are still doctors out there who care, after all."

According to The Star's report, Lieberthal made this blonde, 33-year-old mother of two small boys, addicted to morphine. Her medical records showed she was prescribed 438 units of morphine or Cyclimorph over a period of six months. And this only concerned what was given to her to be administered by injections.

Lieberthal's attorney responded to The Star about Janssens' claims by saying his client refuted her allegations. "Mrs. Janssens is a self-admitted opiate addict and was an addict prior to coming under Dr. Lieberthal's care. She was in fact a Pethidine addict and not a morphine addict and she had been through multiple rehabilitations at many institutions throughout South Africa."

She denied this.

"Our client advises that Mrs. Janssens was discharged from hospital on opiate treatment under the supervision of her husband. It was necessary for her to be weaned off her medication gradually, in order to avoid the ensuring excessive side effects, including fits, which might occur."

This was an out of character concession. Lieberthal was admitting to something which was very much frowned upon by the Medical Council. It did not approve of doctors getting laypeople (husbands, wives, and the like) to supervise or administer strong drugs to patients at home.

Lieberthal claimed Debbie had stolen drugs from a locked cupboard to feed her addiction to opiates. She described this accusation as "outrageous" and called on him to provide the dates and names of the institutions where she had been admitted.

Time does a lot to heal bad memories, but they can easily be revived, so I was not surprised that Debbie did not want to go into detail when I spoke to her years after her story made the papers. "It was a hell of an experience for me that nearly took away my entire life. I have been happy for the last few years, so I don't want to go back there in my mind."

She described some of Lieberthal's remarks as "just bitchy." With its usual lack of concern for patients, the Medical Council never came back to her with the result of her complaint. Putting it mildly, she said, "They were useless."

"Did you ever sue him in court," I asked.

"No. I should have."

She confirmed the correctness of her diary details that had appeared in The Star.

Lieberthal had his admirers. They campaigned for him by sending letters to the papers. The Star published some of them. One was from the man who was prepared to back the surgeon's cause religiously, for better or for worse, no matter what happened. He had been championing the doctor ever since his Medical School days and seemed oblivious to the detrimental evidence that was piling up against his number one surgeon.

Professor Erken wanted to "help to balance the, so far, mostly negative character references in the media". He stressed what a brilliant registrar Lieberthal had been at Wits, adding: "Dr. Lieberthal is at present the most popular teacher in the management of spinal disorders in the Department of Orthopedic Surgery at Wits for both undergraduates and postgraduate students. He is also running, in an honorary capacity, the Children's Spinal Clinic at the Johannesburg Hospital with great efficiency and success."

Another letter was from an M. Arons, who was possibly a doctor or somebody else in the medical field, or perhaps one of Lieberthal's friends. This person's view was that "the hounding of this doctor by the press is despicable, iniquitous and vindictive. His treatment has been nothing short of accusation, trial and conviction by a kangaroo court. What medical expertise and knowledge do his detractors have that entitles them to attack the doctor? Have they sought medical opinions regarding the patients" accusations? Has it crossed their minds that perhaps the complications described by the patients do occur in some cases and are acceptable as a risk of surgery? Any intelligent person who has ever considered or has had a back operation knows that the results are variable and unpredictable, more so than any other surgical discipline."

In the middle of this deluge of publicity that Lieberthal was getting, Thaw got a call at 702 from a young woman. She sounded desperate. "I really need to meet you in person," she said. "It's about Wynne Lieberthal."

"I'd become used to such calls," Thaw told me. "When I first broke the story, our newsroom was snowed under with calls from the surgeon's former patients, so one more was not that significant. Why did I agree to meet this, as yet, unidentified woman? I was intrigued by the cry for help that came across in the sound of her voice. Perhaps she had a new angle."

Walking off to their meeting point at the Breadbasket coffee shop at the Village Walk shopping center, not far from his offices in Sandton, he was blissfully unaware that this would be no ordinary interview.

On his arrival at the rendezvous, an attractive, dark-haired young woman, who was dressed very fashionably, recognized Thaw immediately. She got up from a table to greet him. "At that moment, I sensed something wasn't right. She was incredible composed, which I suppose added to the surrealness of the moment." The second he sat down, the woman, in her early twenties, introduced herself as Kara Lieberthal, Wynne's daughter.

"My stomach flick-flacked into a knot and I swear I felt a nauseous twinge. To her credit, she was as civil as a person, whose family had clearly been deeply affected by the widespread publicity I had set in motion, could be."

In an even tone, devoid of hate or anger, she explained how his constant coverage of her father's past had ruined him. Playing on Thaw's emotions, she took out a framed photograph of her dad with his children. This made Thaw decidedly uneasy, but he maintained his composure.

"To be brutally honest, I felt guilty. Despite the doctor's many verbal attacks on me when I'd been accused of being ruthless and heartless, here I was, being faced with another very sad side of this ongoing drama. According to the surgeon's daughter, I had destroyed not only him, but his entire family as well.

"A story of such intense human interest was always going to hurt somebody. But my reporting on the story was one of the few means available to Lieberthal's former patients to vent their anger about the way they had been treated."

Kara made a passionate plea for him to leave her family alone. He understood how difficult it was for her and her siblings, and realized it must have taken tremendous courage for her to approach him. "I respected her for that. Should I have left the story alone because of the impact it was having on her family? I challenge any journalist to say 'Yes'.

"The meeting lasted about an hour; arguably the most difficult sixty minutes of my career. It fluctuated between a tear-wrenching argument, and a personal attack on me. But, no matter which way I looked at that intensely, uncomfortable experience, the only conclusion that I could come to was that there was only one person she could legitimately blame for all that had happened—Wynne Lieberthal."

Thaw had been working for 702 for just over a year when he had this scoop. He was a 24-year-old news reporter who was "very wet behind the ears" so he neglected to enter the story for any journalistic awards. "Katy said, had I done this, I certainly would have won something." Modestly he added, "I disagree."

Chapter 13

Wounded Surgeon Fights Back

Even though Lieberthal's practice was in free fall, he was not one to give up easily.

He had the resources to fight to clear his name. Screwing people's backs together was extremely lucrative, and screwing them again to cover his mistakes was possibly even more profitable. The money had been pouring in.

The cocky surgeon would not let 702 and The Star get away with the monumental libels they had perpetrated against him. He was convinced he would find a civil court judge who would realize how badly wronged he had been and award him substantial damages. But first, he had to shut them up to salvage the remains of his practice that was running red like an open wound.

His urgent application to stop Talk Radio 702 from defaming him got going in the High Court in Johannesburg in the midst of the storm of publicity. The case began on the Monday and continued for several days throughout that week before Judge Azhar Cashalia came to a decision at the beginning of the following week.

Thaw had covered many stories in the Johannesburg High Court, but he never thought that one of those cases would relate to him. Sitting in the courtroom listening to the doctor's lawyers lash out, threaten and deny he was decidedly nervous. "Was I out of my element?" he wondered. "Had I got in too deep? As I toiled with these insecurities one thing remained crystal clear in my mind: I had uncovered something big, and to be forced back down by a barrage of arrogant legalese would potentially give Dr. Lieberthal the power trip he so craved to fuel his malpractice."

Lieberthal's action was brought against Primedia Broadcasting, the owners of 702. He particularly wanted the station to stop telling the world that he was "Dr. Death" or the "Butcher from Rosebank", and that he had paralyzed his patients, was a drug addict and was not a properly qualified orthopedic surgeon. In his founding affidavit, he claimed that listeners had no doubt that he was the doctor being referred to by 702, even though his name had not been mentioned. At this stage, he was only concerned with 702's first few broadcasts.

"Patients have been phoning me continually about the reports and discussions on 702," he stated. His medical colleagues had also contacted him to enquire about what was being said about him on the radio.

It went without saying that John Robbie's reference to him as "Dr. Death" was denied. "To my knowledge, there are only two individuals throughout history who have been known as Dr. Death, namely Dr. Mengele, a Nazi doctor who tortured innocent children and adults. His acts were atrocious, to say the least. There was also a Dr. Kevorkian in America, who has recently been sentenced to many years' imprisonment. He assisted individuals to commit suicide. Clearly the intention was to convey a meaning that was similar to these two individuals; not competent to practice and a danger to my patients."

In 1999, Dr. Jack Kevorkian was sent to prison for second-degree murder after helping as many as 130 people to take their own lives. He had given them lethal injections while consistently taunting the authorities to take action against him. The 79-year-old retired pathologist was released in 2007 after his sentence was reduced for good behavior and he undertook never to assist in any more suicides.

For somebody trying desperately to avoid publicity, Lieberthal and his legal advisers had evidently not researched media psychology at all. This ghoulish interpretation of why he had been called Dr. Death was a journalist's delight, which could only invite more media interest with the accompanying headlines.

Inevitably, this formed a substantial part of The Star's report of the second day of the application.

Attached to one of Lieberthal's affidavits were copies of certificates to show how qualified he was. These included some given to him for attending various workshops in England and Germany in 1996 and 1997. On one of them, there was the name "Sofamor Danek, Spine Specialists" in the corner.

I was not able to establish who had paid for his trip to the two-day workshop in Hamburg, or whether he paid for this himself. But an orthopedic surgeon told me that he believed Lieberthal used to "work with Sofamor Danek exclusively" and they would more than likely have sent him on a course allied to their instrumentation.

In 2006, Sofamor Danek, makers of spine fusion and artificial discs devices, hit the headlines in America in much the same way Lieberthal had done in South Africa. Its crime was giving kickbacks to doctors to use its products. Sofamor Danek is a division of Medtronic Incorporated, one of the largest medical device manufacturers in the United States. It accounted for 20 percent of the company's 11.3-billion dollar sales in 2005.

Medtronic agreed to pay a $40-million fine to settle the charges against it. A press release issued by the US Department of Justice revealed that between 1998 and 2003 Medtronic paid kickbacks by using sham consulting and royalty agreements and providing lavish trips to desirable locations.

Documents showed that the company made payments of at least $50-million over a four-year period.

The False Claims Act there allows private individuals to file lawsuits on behalf of the US government and collect a share of the money recovered if a Government agency is involved. In this case, it was the Medicare program that was affected.

Whistle blower Jacqueline Peet, a senior travel services manager at Medtronic until 2003, set off this lawsuit. She organized for spine surgeons to attend conferences where the main object was to "induce them through any financial means necessary" to use the company's products. This led to doctors performing unnecessary operations. According to her, Medtronic made a special effort to influence surgeons in training by paying for them to attend over 200 professional meetings a year. The company paid for doctors to do such things as play golf or go snorkeling. When they visited Memphis, they were taken to the Platinum Plus strip club, and the expenses were written off as an "evening at the ballet".

In his effort to silence 702, Lieberthal named Gareth Cliff as the presenter who had first called him the "Butcher of Rosebank". Cliff subsequently moved to the SABC's Radio 5 and was one of the four judges in the fourth and fifth season of M-Net television's Idols pop star competition. He also had his own chat show on M-Net television.

Katy Katopodis was denounced for a news bulletin she read that labeled Lieberthal as having paralyzed many of his patients, being a drug addict, and not being properly qualified.

He maintained the statements made about him on 702 were totally false and defamatory. They gave listeners the impression that he was not worthy to practice as a doctor; did not follow the Hippocratic Oath; was a danger to the public; partook in illegal activities and caused death and anguish to his patients.

In the first week of the case, the documents submitted by both sides were piling up to voluminous proportions. The ones from Yusuf Abramjee, Radio 702's manager, outlining the station's defense ran to 219 pages. And then, there was Lieberthal's sworn version of what he believed happened. It was wishful thinking on behalf of the doctor if he thought this public debate was suddenly, like Omo, going to make his dirty washing whiter than white, even if he won his case.

Abramjee described the terrible experiences of various people who had consulted Lieberthal. To back his allegations, Duncan Turner of Webber Wentzel Bowens, 702's attorneys, had taken statements or spoken to them.

Mrs. Arlette Buisansky ran a stable on the outskirts of Johannesburg and taught riding when she saw Lieberthal in June 2000. Her neck had been injured in a car accident 23 years earlier, but she emphasized that she had not gone to see Lieberthal about her neck, but because she was having back ache.

He showed her on the x-rays that she had spurs on her cervical spine, which, if not removed, would cause her to lose all movement in her upper body, especially her arms. "This scared the hell out of me, as my job is a very physical one, aside from not wanting to end up paralyzed. Dr. Lieberthal was so charming and convincing that I believed him," she related in a four-page letter.

Lieberthal told her he would fuse vertebrae in her neck with the use of a cage, which, he said, was a method that was new to the country. She was in so much pain that she went ahead with the operation at the Rosebank Clinic.

Instead of being back to normal and able to drive within a week, as Lieberthal had promised, she endured months of agony and was confined to bed for many weeks, unable to do anything. A year after the operation she was still taking pain control tablets and was still suffering from neck spasms, vibrations, and hands that were shaking so much her handwriting was illegible.

"There were days when I was totally dysfunctional. My speech and memory were hopeless. On those days, all I could do was to stay in bed, unable to do the simplest of things, let alone work. I had long ago stopped going to gym as this put my muscles into more spasms."

One of the doctors in her GP practice referred her to Dr. Carle van Heerden, a neurosurgeon, because she was feeling so terrible. He examined her, looked at all her x-rays and concluded that Lieberthal should not have operated on her, as it was virtually impossible to get to the base of the spurs without damaging the spinal cord. Neurologist Dr. David Isaacs agreed with Van Heerden's opinion.

Her physical condition was still not even close to what it was before the neck fusion was done. "I feel that it was very unethical of Dr. Lieberthal to do an unnecessary operation on me by scaring me with paralysis," her letter ended.

In his defense, Lieberthal declared himself "shocked" at Abramjee's claim that Buisansky had been "permanently disabled" after he operated on her, when there was nothing in her letter to indicate this. He denied her "false and unfounded allegations" against him and stated, "She has never complained to me and to the best of my knowledge neither to the HPCSA".

Turner had a telephone conversation with George St George, a blind man whose wife Denise was a receptionist at the Rosebank Clinic when Lieberthal operated on his back. St George said that Lieberthal was intent on surgery from the outset. He was asked to sign some papers, but as he could not see, he did not know what he was signing.

He had since been under the care of Dr. Frank Snyckers, a neurosurgeon who had attempted to fix the problem Lieberthal created. But he was still partially paralyzed, as his legs collapsed when he tried to walk. "Dr. Lieberthal has ruined my life," he told Turner.

In his replying affidavit, Lieberthal said that St George was over 60-year-old when he saw him. He had been treated for a considerable time for numerous psychiatric disorders. Lieberthal used him as a case study at a lecture he gave with two other orthopedic surgeons at the Johannesburg Hospital.

"St George was examined by me, Dr. Rodrigues and Dr. Majusa and, in addition thereto, a discussion ensued with the trainee surgeons relating to St George's problem," Lieberthal revealed.

"He was diagnosed with lumbar instability and each one of the surgeons concurred on the treatment, namely lumbar stabilization, being a lumbar spine fusion."

St George initially got scared after being admitted to hospital for the operation. He discharged himself. However, because of the pain he was having, he returned later and had the fusion.

"Following a successful and uneventful surgical procedure, St George convalesced in the ward for a few days and was thereafter discharged," Lieberthal went on. "There was no paralysis, whatsoever. He never complained to me, nor has his wife complained that I did anything wrong. In any event, I respectfully submit that I did nothing wrong and attended to St George in a proper manner as was required at the time."

I spoke to St George's wife on the pavement outside the front gate of the townhouse complex in the Ridgeway suburb of Southern Johannesburg where she lived. A good-looking woman in her early sixties with her hair streaked with grey, she showed her reluctance to be interviewed by not inviting me into her apartment.

With a pained expression she said, "I don't think I want to get involved because I worked with Dr. Lieberthal at the Rosebank Clinic. It's such a sad story, and it brings back so many bad memories. My husband really relied on him. I had three nervous breakdowns after my husband died and I don't want to go back over all that stuff."

Her Italian husband was a diesel mechanic who went blind overnight at the age of 45. He died aged 63 and his wife retired from her job at the Clinic two months later. The couple had been divorced for years but, as they continued to live together, nobody was aware of this as she still referred to him as her husband. She had evidently stayed with him, as she was the breadwinner.

"He was a very active person who wanted to work, but he couldn't because he was blind," she said. "This resulted in him having major depression. Then he fell and cracked a vertebra in his back. Dr. Lieberthal did the op, and all the screws fell out. Then we had to have it redone by Dr. Snyckers. If he had gone to Dr. Snyckers in the first place, maybe my husband would still be alive. I don't know.

"Afterwards, people came to us to ask my husband if he wanted to sue Lieberthal. I said "No" and my husband didn't want to, either. It wouldn't have improved his health and his quality of life was so poor anyway, we just left it.

"You know the medical fraternity will not run each other down. You can say what you like and they won't say, oh he did this or he did that. I mean, why would you have to have an operation redone if the screws didn't fall out?"

Doctors doing nothing about their wayward colleagues concerned me, so I said, "As you say that's part of the problem…"

"Um."

"… that the medical fraternity sticks together. They can see Jon Abbott doing rubbishy operations for years and they do nothing about it."

"Well, this is the thing and even now it's still going on."

"I've spoken to quite a lot of people who said Lieberthal was absolutely charming in the beginning. But once it was clear there was a big problem, they couldn't get hold of him. He just disappeared."

"No, no, no, I could always get hold of him," she said, with honest impartiality.

"Even after there were problems?" I persisted.

"Yes. But of course he wouldn't tell you there were problems. My husband had so many other problems it was difficult to say what the problem was, but with his back there was no doubt. The x-rays proved that. When I told him my husband wanted to see Dr. Snyckers for a second opinion, he said 'That's fine'. He even gave me a report on the op he did. He was very nice about it. No, I always found him a very nice person." I had managed to speak to her just in time. She was planning to go and live in Canada with her daughter, as she no longer had any relatives in South Africa.

Abramjee's next example was 81-year-old Mrs. Margaret Buchanan. She had been in the Queenshaven Retirement Village in the South of Johannesburg for several years. This was established by the Johannesburg Coronation Foundation to commemorate the coronation of Queen Elizabeth II. It could take around 400 old people. There, the resident doctor was Lieberthal's long-time friend, Dr. Steven Brower. He held a daily clinic at the village and treated the residents whenever necessary.

When Buchanan complained to Brower about her backache, he sent her to see Lieberthal in August 2002. If she had problems before she saw the surgeon Brower had recommended, they were nothing compared to what happened afterwards.

According to Abramjee: "A statement from Mr. Derrick Tabbert, the grandson of Mrs. Buchanan, catalogues his grandmother's treatment at the applicant's hands that has left her paralyzed below her waist." The statement was taken from Tabbert because his grandmother was too old and infirm to give one herself.

Abramjee's allegations certainly raised Lieberthal's ire. "It is disingenuous, scurrilous, malicious, and defamatory to allege that my treatment has left Buchanan paralyzed," the surgeon retaliated. He did a caudal and facet joint block on Buchanan, which involved injecting cortisone into her spine. At all times he had made it clear to her that the treatment was remedial rather than a cure.

"We met with Dr. Lieberthal directly after the operation," Derrick wrote in a letter of complaint he and his mother, Jean, sent to the Health Professions Council. "He told us that the operation had been successful because he had removed a blood clot from the area and the spinal cord was pulsating."

Lieberthal's window-dressing optimism turned out to be very wide of the mark. "My mother went from the sick bay at Queenshaven to the frail care, and she never got up again," Jean told me. "She died eight months after first being admitted to hospital, having been bedridden since then. She had been a fun-loving, happy person until she went to see Lieberthal."

A blonde, homely Scot, Jean was running a laboratory and scientific glass-blowing business. She had inherited it from her husband Dieter, who died of cancer aged 63.

As if her mother's experience with Lieberthal was not enough to distress anybody, Jean had to argue with Brower over what had caused her mother's death. "Dr. Brower said to me, 'What must I put on the death certificate?' I replied, 'I don't believe it, you're the bloody doctor'. He said, 'A stroke?' and I said, 'She had pneumonia'. He ended up putting "natural causes" on the certificate."

She and her son got an acknowledgement from the HPCSA that their complaint had been received, and that was the last they heard from this uncaring body.

Another litany of pain Abramjee produced for Lieberthal to answer was in Ian Collet's statement. This referred to "15 different surgical procedures done on him by the applicant and the dangerous situation created by leaking spinal fluid because the applicant had not fixed the prosthetic screws properly".

All this was done over a 20-month period in 2001 and 2002 and, as Collet's condition was as bad as ever, he changed to Dr. Snyckers. Snyckers told him he would have to undergo further surgery because the instrumentation Lieberthal had put in had come loose.

Collet told Turner that a neurologist who tested him concluded he had a pinched nerve in his spine. Lieberthal undertook to release this to relieve the pain he was suffering. He said the operation would take about an hour and Collet would be able to go home within two days. This promise turned out to be as empty as the exhausted medical aid funds of many of his patients after he had finished with them.

When Collet woke up after one of his operations, he was in intensive care. Next to his bed was a packet containing eight screws marked 07.5; two metal bars connected by a crossbar looking like a rugby goal post and nuts for the end of the screws, and when Lieberthal saw Collet in ICU he told him, "When I opened up your back, I noticed that everything had fallen apart so I had to replace the entire mechanism again".

That operation was done in July, even though Lieberthal had replaced one set of screws with a new lot six months earlier. As the wound would not heal, it had to be surgically cleaned a few days later. On his thirteenth day in hospital, Lieberthal saw Collet and issued an instruction for him to be discharged the next day, but before he was due to leave Collet told nurses that he was concerned because the dressing on the wound was still wet. They assured him that his surgeon was satisfied that he could go home.

Hospital nurses could do nothing unless a doctor authorized it. They were never allowed to suggest that the gods of medicine, especially a perfect one like Lieberthal, might have made a mistake.

Later that afternoon, while Collet was lying in bed at home, the sheet was flooded by fluid draining from his wound. He called Lieberthal, who told him to return to the Rosebank Clinic immediately. On the telephone, Lieberthal said he would operate the following day to patch the leak.

Collet's father drove him back to the clinic where the leak was successfully closed, and a week later he was discharged from hospital once again.

Nobody was going to pin any of Collet's bad experiences on Lieberthal that was clear from his affidavit. He resorted to splitting hairs to try and make his treatment of Collet appear a lot better than it was being made out to be by Abramjee. "There were not 15 different surgical procedures. There were five, the remainder being conservative treatment options, which are not surgical procedures," his repudiation went on.

As he had done previously, Lieberthal put the blame on other people, including Collet himself. "I did not create a dangerous situation because I had not fixed prosthetic screws properly. The spinal leak was due to the myelogram done by the radiologist." This is a procedure where iodine is injected into a specific area to highlight on x-rays anything that might be wrong.

But if the dates (they were not disputed by Lieberthal) given by Collet for the 15 procedures were correct, then the radiologist was entirely blameless because the myelogram was done on 25 September, more than a month after Lieberthal had closed the leak.

It was Collet's fault the implants failed, the doctor maintained, because he had returned to work despite being told not to, did nothing to reduce his excessive weight, and was a poorly controlled diabetic.

"I was not the first surgeon who saw Collet," Lieberthal claimed. "In fact, he had multiple surgical procedures by Dr. Frank Snykers prior to consulting me."

An operation that had "disastrous consequences for a patient" that Abramjee raised involved Yossie Danino. At that stage, he was busy suing Lieberthal in the High Court for R863 000, although the case had not yet been finalized.

In the particulars of Danino's claim, according to Abramjee, it was recorded that Mrs. Danino observed Lieberthal did the back operation on her husband when he, Lieberthal, had a broken arm and "therefore presumably with one hand". Lieberthal was negligent because he operated on the wrong disc and failed to diagnose the thrombosis that developed in Danino's left leg.

Lieberthal used the sub judice excuse for not giving his version of what happened when he treated Danino. His attorneys, MacRobert Incorporated, advised him not to go into details as that case was still pending. However, he denied the allegations being made against him.

Denise Vos, the sister who worked in the theatre at the Rosebank Clinic for many years, told me, "Wynne was actually a slim little fellow. Then he started going to the gym. He was putting on muscle like you can't believe. I said, 'Gee, where did you get all these muscles from?' He was really hitting the gym big time, but he was doing too much; using too many weights or something, and it went off like a gunshot. His humerus just fractured."

This happened a year or two before all the publicity blew up in the media. "Then he did the wrong thing," she continued. "He tried to operate with one arm."

"How can you operate with one arm in a sling?" I asked.

"He had been told he had to rest his arm for about six weeks and not do anything. But he came back to work. Other doctors were very upset about this. They felt it really isn't the thing to do to come into theatre and your patient's lying there and you've got one arm in a sling. He did have another surgeon with him and he supervised the operation. But they felt he should never have done that."

Once again I said to myself: If there were doctors who felt what he was doing was wrong, why didn't they do something about it, like reporting him to the Health Professions Council?

"That arm never healed properly," she said. "I think he got osteomyelitis." It was an infection in the bone which was difficult to cure.

His law firm of MacRobert Incorporated acted for the Medical Protection Society so Lieberthal would probably not have had to dip into his own pocket to fund his defense of Danino's claim or to pay any damages if he lost. This was the same firm of lawyers, now with a shortened name, that Brower asked for help when I questioned him. They had the lucrative job of dealing with all the Societies' cases.

As it happened, Lieberthal did lose, but that was some time after his application to silence 702. Danino walked away with an out of court settlement of R300 000.

An Israeli, who came to South Africa in 1986, Danino told me that at the age of 20, he fell down a 15 meter high bank during maneuvers in Lebanon while he was in the Israeli army. He had no immediate problems, but gradually his back began bothering him.

On a trip to Sun City in January 2002, he did a twisting motion as he picked up his young son. A sudden excruciating pain in his back shot down both legs. It was so bad that he collapsed on the floor. He was attended to by the casino's paramedics. His wife drove him back to Johannesburg and the next morning he was seen by Lieberthal in his rooms.

The alarming tale of incompetence that occurred after that was revealed in the court documents of Danino's case. When the color of his left foot changed from blue to purple, Lieberthal admitted him to the Rosebank Clinic. In agony, he arrived in a wheelchair.

Lieberthal diagnosed a slipped disc that was affecting Danino's nerves, and this, in turn, was possibly compromising the blood flow to his leg. He removed a damaged disc and did a fusion. Over the next few days, Danino complained to Lieberthal about the pain, the lack of feeling, the coldness, and the unhealthy color of his left leg and foot. On three separate occasions, Lieberthal assured him that everything was fine and that the nerve could take up to six months to regenerate.

Danino's and his wife's doubts about Lieberthal's competency probably saved him from losing his leg. His wife took him to the Linksfield Clinic, where he was seen by a cardiac physician and other specialists. They discovered he had no pulse in his left foot because of clots in his arteries from the knee downwards. An operation was performed to remove these, but as one of them re-formed, he had to have another procedure to get rid of that one.

In a medico-legal report done for Danino's claim by neurosurgeon Dr. Gian Marus, he referred to Lieberthal's other serious bungle. The x-ray showed Lieberthal operated on the wrong level. "He considered the L3/4 disc space as the L4/5 space; thus removing a normal disc. The consequences are that the L3/4 segment, which was anatomically normal, has been infringed upon by a discectomy and has been fused. Luckily, the L4/5 segment where the disc sequestration had taken place was also operated upon and the disc was removed, thus decompressing the nerve root. However, this movement segment has not been fused. So, with the adjacent fusion, it is likely to aggravate the mechanical stresses on it, giving rise to his present back symptoms and impairment."

Lieberthal's account, together with that of the Clinic, came to R78 066. Dr. Marus described Lieberthal's fees as "excessive" for the lumbar fusion that was performed.

What really astonished me was what Danino told me about Lieberthal and the condition of his back when I saw him five years after the treatment that had been the subject of his legal action.

"My back op was a success," he said, smiling broadly.

"Oh, was it?" I replied, finding this hard to believe.

"*Ja.* I have been good for the last four years. My back's never been better my whole life since the fusion. What he did for me was great. Yes, he had a broken arm when he did my op. But you know what? If he had operated with two fingers, he did the job for me. What can I say, this is the facts. Today I wouldn't take that money because I don't think I deserved it. But maybe I did because of the leg and the suffering. I could have lost my foot maybe, I don't know."

"You were very lucky," I remarked.

"Listen, he had good hands. He had a very good brain. But I believe he became greedy for money and there were obvious implications for that."

A fit-looking man in his early fifties, Danino could not stop praising the final result of what Lieberthal did for him. "What happened around it was not right. I got paid for my suffering, and whatever. I don't have to go to another doctor to do any other procedure for now. Looking at the whole thing I could have been on the wrong side, as well, but I'm on the right side, thank God."

Danino was even able to play golf, a sport that had caused serious back problems for some of the world's top professionals. He had a seven handicap. About six months after his operation, somebody from The Star interviewed him and they took his picture. "Where did they find me? On the golf course." That amused him and he laughed before saying, "On the 14th or whatever. The reporter actually came to the Houghton golf course."

As the case proceeded, The Star did not let up. Collet's revelations in the court documents appeared under a massive headline "Knives out for surgeon." A mountain of a man who looked like a Sumo wrestler, he was pictured in his hospital bed holding up a packet of the screws that had been removed from his back. According to The Star, the number of complaints against Lieberthal that had been made to the Medical Council had now reached 19. And his aggrieved former patients were invited by the HPCSA to lodge any complaints they had as soon as possible.

702's main witness, of course, was Cooper. It was difficult, if not impossible, for any doctor to defend an allegation of incompetence if he had left part of a razor-sharp scalpel in somebody's back. In his affidavit, Lieberthal dealt extensively with what Cooper had to say about him. Mostly he denied having done anything wrong, although he admitted to leaving the tip of that scalpel blade behind. Before he closed the wound, he attempted to retrieve it. "This was not possible," he claimed. The tip could not be felt with a rougeur, so it was elected to leave it in the disc space and to monitor it on serial x-rays. It was approximately three millimeters long and about as wide.

"At no time was the fact of the blade tip remaining in the disc space kept from him and I did not tell him it would never move."

He maintained that, when he operated on Cooper for the first time to close the fluid leak in the dura, he found it had been caused by a spicule of bone. He removed this and sealed the leak. Once again, he blamed his patient for what happened next. The leak restarted. "Cooper knew that he was not to get out of bed, but he did so, in spite of my instructions," was Lieberthal's angry comment.

As the leak did not heal properly, another operation became necessary, but by that time Cooper had decided to ask Dr. George Zwonnikoff, a neurosurgeon, for a second opinion. According to Lieberthal, Zwonnikoff was not prepared to take on Cooper as a patient and that was when he moved to Dr. Hoffman, who repaired the leak.

When it came to refuting under oath, other so-called "libelous" allegations made on 702, Lieberthal once again showed that sworn statements were meaningless to him. One caller got a special mention. "I do not know who this alleged patient is. It strikes me as bizarre that this individual could have undergone 24 back operations by me and be paralyzed and want to remain anonymous."

It was even more bizarre that he did not know who she was, yet I managed to find her five years down the line. And what she told me showed the doctor up for what he was—a habitual liar even when he was under oath.

Pamela Bekink was living in a rundown house in a poor part of the Johannesburg suburb of Rosettenville. She struggled to walk on crutches, and when she was not lying down, she found it less painful to move about the house on all fours, on more or less the same level as her three dogs. Her problems began when she was injured at work.

She had documents to show that between August 1997 and September 2000, Lieberthal had done 24 back operations on her. She was not, strictly speaking, paralyzed, however she was badly crippled.

"I understand that when all this blew up about Lieberthal in the papers and on 702, you phoned the radio station," I said.

Lying on her lounge couch, this 62-year-old divorcee replied, "Yes, that very day. I was still a listener of 702 at that time, a very staunch listener. That day that it broke on the radio, I listened, I listened, listened some more. I thought, 'Could it be?' Let me phone. I dialed the number, and I got through."

"Well, what did you say on the radio?"

"First of all, I asked the lady who the doctor was, and she said she couldn't say. Why was I inquiring? I said, 'Well there was also a doctor in a similar capacity who had done 24 operations on me'. When she asked who the doctor was, I told her it was Dr. Lieberthal, and she replied, 'Well, that's the doctor'." She moved awkwardly to another position to try and relieve her pain. "All of a sudden, another phone got picked up, and I was questioned about why I had so many operations and so on."

"Was this broadcast on the air?" I asked.

"Yes." Indignantly she continued, "And on the next news, my damned voice came over. They didn't give my name, but I've got such a distinctive voice, any monkey can recognize it. I was so blooming mad that they put that tape on and both he and his secretary heard it on the radio."

The same day he phoned her, demanding to know what she thought she was saying on the radio.

"'I don't know what you are talking about', I told him. And when he said, 'You've just been on the news', I said, 'It must have been somebody else'.

"He was very stern. I thought, 'Oh God is he going to take me to court. What have I said?' I didn't condemn him. I didn't say anything I shouldn't have said. All I said was that I was similar to these other people who had had all these operations. Then I started cross-examining myself because I didn't know what was going to happen next. So I said to myself I must listen to the news and see if it's going to come again. And it did, about two or three times that day."

"Did he ever contact you again?"

"No, not until some time later after I sent a complaint to the Medical Council. They sent him a copy of it and he phoned me to ask my reason for sending it."

Lieberthal's perjured himself still further in his affidavit by saying, "I emphatically deny that I underwent drug rehabilitation treatment in approximately 1991." That had been what a caller had claimed. It was hard to understand what Lieberthal was thinking when he made this statement under oath, because he knew that there was extensive documentary evidence that showed that the caller had been perfectly right.

Another beef Lieberthal had with 702 was that it was only allowing one side of the story to be aired–the bad one. "I am aware of the names of numerous individuals who telephoned 702 to give positive comments relating to me, but the respondent refused to air their calls," he protested.

"Ariel Isaacson had to tell the show producer that he wanted to complain about me before they would put him on the show. Ariel, however, did not complain about me," his affidavit went on.

He then listed 18 people, who, he said, had good things to say about him, but were not given the chance by 702.

Maliza Booysens, the girl who had nothing but praise for Lieberthal for saving her life, castigated Beeld, The Star, and 702, for not wanting to use her story because it was a positive one.

Her mother Leonie sent a facsimile to 702, giving a rundown of the way Lieberthal helped her daughter when other doctors had failed. "I was really shocked that 702 could broadcast such nonsense," she told the station. "Dr. Lieberthal is for us an angel that the Lord sent after much prayer. Now it's my turn to get down on my knees to pray that all his supporters will contact the radio station to show that they stand by him. In all my years that I have known Dr. Lieberthal, I have never known him to behave in an unprofessional manner towards my family or any other person who we have referred to him. I personally know of a doctor in Alberton who had 14 patients die in five years and nothing gets done about that."

When judgment day arrived, Lieberthal must have been watching His Honor with a mixture of hope and apprehension, trying to gauge which way the case was going to go. Like most judgments, the Judge's introduction and review of the evidence gave no hint of the final outcome.

He said that, since the matter first came to court, both 702 and The Star continued to give the increasing stream of allegations prominence in their news reports. And, although Lieberthal had given notice that he intended taking legal action against this newspaper, it was not party to these proceedings.

Listening to the judgment, Lieberthal's emotions must have gone up and down like a Yo-Yo. The Judge said 702 contended that its defense was truth; in the public interest and fair comment. Setting out the approach the courts had adopted in striking a balance between freedom of speech and the protection of a person's reputation, he relied on an earlier case. This involved the Argus Company, the former owners of The Star.

In that case Judge Corbett concluded: "The right of free expression enjoyed by all persons, including the press, must yield to the individual's right which is just as important not to be unlawfully defamed. I emphasize the word 'unlawfully', for in striving to achieve an equitable balance between the right to speak your mind and the right not to be harmed by what others say about you, the law has devised a number of defenses, such as fair comment; justification such as truth and the public interest and privilege which, if successfully invoked, renders lawful the publication of matter which is prima facie defamatory.

"Ultimately there can be no justification for the publication of untruths and members of the press should not be left with the impression that they have a license to lower the standards of care which must be observed before a defamatory matter is published in a newspaper."

Returning to the details of Lieberthal's case, Cachalia said, "There can be no doubt that the allegations concerning negligence against the applicant, including gross negligence, which led to paralysis in a few cases, are defamatory in the sense that the statements tend to lower the applicant in the estimation of ordinary right-thinking or intelligent members of society. From the nature and tone of the allegations it is apparent that 702, has on occasions exaggerated the extent of the applicant's alleged negligence. For example, one news report alleges that former patients claim the applicant 'left scalpels in their backs', while another one alleges that 'the doctor left scores of patients paralyzed'. No factual basis has been laid for these allegations. In some cases, the "facts" put forward by 702 do not support any allegation of negligence.

"Despite these shortcomings I am not persuaded that 702 will not be able to refute the charge relating to the applicant's competency as an orthopedic surgeon, or the particular charge that he 'paralyzed his patients'. It would not have to prove every allegation provided that it is able to prove that the general charge is substantially true or at least that it is reasonable in the sense that the facts relied upon were properly sourced. They are clearly in the public interest."

Delivering Lieberthal a body blow that must have paled even this arrogance specialist he said, "Having regard to the totality of the evidence, I am led to the conclusion that the Defences of truth and public benefit, reasonableness and fair comment on matters of public interest are sustainable."

Giving Lieberthal another glimmer of hope, he continued, "But the inquiry does not end there. The applicant contends that the balance of convenience favours him as he has no alternative remedy and that he will have difficulty in determining the damages suffered as a result of the publication of these statements.

"It is true that damages in defamation actions are difficult to prove and often no amount of monetary compensation can adequately compensate the damage to a person's reputation, particularly after having been subjected to the allegations which the applicant has faced over the last week and indeed continues to face.

"But there are factors which favour 702 as well. As regards the fact that there is no alternative remedy, it is clear that 702 has afforded the applicant an opportunity to give his side of the story right from the beginning. The applicant declines to use this avenue. Now that the matter is in the public domain an interdict by its very nature will not be an effective remedy. Indeed, it would amount to a form of ineffective censorship."

He quoted from Burchell's The Law of Defamation where the author said, "The public interest is better served by continuing debate through rebuttal than by compulsorily bringing it to an end."

Regarding the references to Lieberthal as "Dr. Death," "the Butcher of Rosebank," and not being properly qualified, 702 had given an undertaking not to repeat them after the court had indicated its displeasure regarding the use of these descriptions. For this reason, he was not going to grant Lieberthal an interdict to silence 702 on this score.

The allegation that Lieberthal was a drug addict then came up. "One would have expected the denial to go beyond merely stating that he did not undergo treatment in 1991, but not too much revolves around this. It is clear from the context in which it was used that a reference to his drug addiction seriously calls into question his competence, precision and clarity of thought.

"As a general principle, it is for the public benefit that the truth about the character or the conduct of individuals should be made known. But the fact that an individual may have transgressed in the past does not necessarily make such transgressions relevant to his present true character. Nor, might I add, do such transgressions have any relevance to his competence to practice professionally at present.

"Even if I assume that the applicant's denials of drug addiction are false, in my view his alleged transgressions are entirely irrelevant to any discussion on his present competence as an orthopedic surgeon. I should add that drug addiction is not a crime, and the rehabilitation of drug addicts should be encouraged and not become a matter of public opprobrium."

He ruled that 702 should cease calling the doctor a drug addict or referring to any past treatment he might have had.

Most importantly for 702 and the media in general, Cachalia upheld the station's right to go on exposing Lieberthal's "disastrous shortcomings."

The result was a double blow for Lieberthal because the judge decided that, as 702 had been "substantially successful", he would have to pay the radio station's costs. These, together with his own legal fees, must have been very substantial.

702 issued a statement saying it was "delighted" with the result and Abramjee added, "It is not only a victory for 702 Talk Radio but also for our listeners and the media. We wish to reiterate that Dr. Lieberthal is more than welcome to respond to the numerous allegations of gross negligence leveled against him. We are prepared to give him one hour on any show—live and unedited."

Encouraged by its court room success, the news editor Katopodis said, "We are continuing with our investigative reports. If and when more details become available, we will report them. It is after all in the interest of the public."

The Star trumpeted the result under the headline: "Court denies doctor's attempt at media gag." Other headlines that appeared in the paper immediately before and after the judgement included: "Docs queue of irate patients keeps growing"; "Doctor made me an addict—housewife"; "Minister of Health alerted to Lieberthal" and "Patients, peers line up to finger Lieberthal."

The day after he had been branded a loser by the Judge, Lieberthal finally decided to grant The Star an interview. He was seen by reporters Alisha Kalideen and Gill Gifford.

Their account headlined: "Surgeon cut up about 'trial by media'", quoted Lieberthal as saying, "It has been devastating. I've had every single theatre list cancelled from the time the news broke. Consultations form only a small part of a surgeon's income. Today should be theatre day, but I don't have a single case."

Sitting with his attorney Graeme Krawitz, he complained that he had been found guilty and crucified by the media. This had made him afraid of driving his car with his children in it because of the newspaper sellers on the streets with banner headlines referring to him.

He always adopted a conservative approach to his patients before resorting to surgery. Most of them came to him as a last resort because 90 percent had previously been operated on by other doctors.

Krawitz said his client would not accept 702's offer to give his side of the story because, "We feel he will further subject himself to trial by media."

Only a few months elapsed before Lieberthal's threats became a reality. In November 2002, he fired off summonses against The Star and Primedia. He might not have been able to shut them up, but these organizations were now going to have to pay big time for embarrassing him publicly and decimating his very profitable practice.

It was imaginative stuff. The figures he arrived at were what most people only dream about if they were to win a lottery. It was the doctor's version of journalistic license because the ridiculous part was that the summonses admitted that his lotto numbers were just optimistic guesses.

The Star was the first to be lined up in his sights.

Some of The Star stories that had particularly peeved him included: "Patient to sue surgeon who left a scalpel in his back"; "The untouchable surgeon who botched this man's op is still at it despite a litany of complaints over eight years"; "An absolute farce; she is bent over and doubled up in pain. The man she blames for ruining her life walks free"; "I was screwed. More and more ex-patients file complaints against surgeon", and "My ordeal. Mother accuses doctor and tells of six operations and morphine addiction. Doctor denies claims and says she stole drugs from a locked cupboard."

His list of what people would have thought about him as a result of The Star's articles was more or less a repeat of what he had put in his summons when he wanted to silence 702. It was all that highly exaggerated stuff about him ruining people's lives; being dishonest; not following the Hippocratic Oath, and so on.

The price that he put on six of The Star's reports to make him feel better was R200 000 a time. To this, he added another R10-million for loss of profits, making a handy R11.2-million.

Primedia got the next summons for what had been said about him on the radio and on 702"s internet site.

The spoken word appeared to have got up his nose far more than the written one because, not only did he list Primedia as the first defendant, but he also named six of 702"s staff members, who were presenters of their own shows or had read news items about the notorious doctor. They were; Robbie, Cliff, Katopodis, Thaw, Nomzamo Khumalo and Francis Hurd. Strangely, Noeleen Maholwana-Sangqu fell outside his net despite having hosted that hour-long talk show that mentioned him numerous times, if not by name then by inference.

The damage done to him on 16 occasions by the people he named, as well as other unspecified individuals, was again valued at R200 000 each. Then he upped the total to R13.2-million, with his standard R10-million for "special patrimonial loss" because of reduced profits. This special loss was a very generous guess. The give-away was in the court documents, where it was explained that "the precise amount is not presently known to the Plaintiff, but is estimated in the sum of R10-million."

Primedia's legal team described Lieberthal's allegations as: "Vague and embarrassing in that they, and the particulars of claim as a whole, do not contain factual averments to sustain the recoverability on any delictual basis of the damages set out in the particulars of claim."

The surgeon's huge ego was getting the better of him. He was behaving like many armies throughout history. Fighting on many fronts was stretching his resources to the limit. Something had to give. With the legal process habitually trundling on so slowly, it was going to take a year or two.

Chapter 14

Adding Insult To Injury

Like Maliza Booysen and her parents, Mariskca du Plessis and her mother Ester will also remember Lieberthal for the rest of their lives. They will remember him as the surgeon who so drastically changed Mariskca's entire future when she was just entering her teens with every hope of an improvement in her bedeviled life.

Mariskca was a happy little girl, even though her father was far from being an ideal dad. All things considered, there was nothing to suggest that, at the age of three, she could not look forward to a completely normal life.

Midway through her third year she was dealt a most vicious hand. It was a billion to one chance that could only be described as the worst possible case of unbelievable bad luck. She just happened to be in the wrong place, through no fault of her own, when it went off.

Ester's first husband was Shaun Ludek. They had two children, Mariskca and Sane`, who was two years younger than her sister. The family lived West of Johannesburg at Westonaria, among what had been some of the richest gold mines in the world.

Ludek, an only child, had a long history of heavy drinking and unpredictable, violent behavior. His marriage to Ester was a very stormy affair. This had such an effect on his two children that, in later years, they refused to acknowledge him as their father.

Shaun was working on a gold mine when it happened. He was also doing periodic air force camps as part of his National Service. He had been home on leave and had planned to hitch-hike back to base. When he didn't get a lift after waiting at the roadside for a while, he returned home, intending to go the next day.

He always kept his 9 millimeter pistol loaded when he hitch-hiked because he believed getting lifts could be dangerous. When he got back to his house, the rest of the family were milling about in the kitchen.

"As he walked in, he took his pistol out to put it on top of the cupboard," Ester told me. "The hammer got hooked on his army clothes and BANG, a shot went off. We didn't realize what had happened at first. Then we saw our baby was bleeding. Mariskca had been shot."

The family rallied round. Mariskca was taken to Krugersdorp Hospital, where she was admitted. She went into theatre that night and transferred to the spinal unit at the H.F. Verwoerd Hospital in Pretoria the following morning, where she remained for the next year and a half.

The bullet from her father's gun had gone through the right side of Mariskca's chest and had come out on the left side of her stomach. It devastated her insides to such an extent that it was a miracle she survived. She lost a kidney. The bullet passed so close to her spinal cord that, although it did not sever it, enough nerve damage was done to paralyze both her legs.

To make matters worse for Mariskca, her environment at home was like a horror movie with her father as the unpredictable, vicious brute. Nobody knew what he was going to do next.

Shaun couldn't face up to the fact that he had shot his baby girl, even though it was clearly an accident. He reacted in a way that was impossible to justify, particularly to a little girl who was being made to feel that the accident was all her fault.

"He was really a dog," said Ester. "He was a psychopath, actually. He felt very guilty about what had happened, but he couldn't handle it. So he couldn't stand to be near Mariskca." For this reason, she decided to let her go and live with Ella, her grandmother, to protect her from her father's abuse. "It was ugly. 'I'll break your bloody neck, you little bitch' were the kind of things he said to her. He was a very bad person. He didn't knock her about, but he did with me."

In time, Mariskca's condition improved. The feeling in her legs began to return. The plucky little girl started crawling and, at the age of six, she was walking with crutches. After that, her general health was excellent, but she was plagued by muscle spasms in her legs. Between 1993 and 1997, she had five or six muscle release operations at the Johannesburg Hospital. "It was a terrible time for her, but she was very brave," her mother said.

"My husband was always threatening to commit suicide when he got drunk. At a certain stage, the welfare people told me that unless I divorced him, they would not allow Mariskca back into my custody." In 1992, she divorced Ludek to get Mariskca back.

Getting rid of the well-built, six foot tall psychopath was not going to be easy. He kept bouncing back, usually with unpleasant consequences. More abuse was followed by groveling apologies.

Confiding in me as though I was a close relative, Ester said, "On one of the occasions that he phoned and asked me to take him back, I refused. Next minute, I got a call from somebody to tell me to come and take him to hospital because he's taken an overdose of pills. That kind of thing happened often." Another time he walked into her home when she had someone with her. "Who's this?" he asked in a threatening tone. And when she replied, "A friend," he got aggressive and told the guy, "What are you doing with my wife? Bugger off." The man got so scared he disappeared in a hurry.

"This is how Shaun was. He once put his pistol to my head. He was going to shoot me and then the kids. He would also hit me and lock me in a room for hours. It was mental and physical torture."

She took two jobs to support herself and the children. In the daytime, she worked for Armadillo Concepts, a firm that manufactured motor accessories. At night, she sold armed response contracts for a security company. Mariskca was at the Hope School for disabled children in Johannesburg, where she was nicknamed Mickey. It was a semi-government establishment. This meant her mother still had to pay some fees, which she could ill afford.

"It all got too much for me, so I decided Shaun was not going to get away with not paying maintenance any longer. I decided to go through the Magistrate's Court in Pretoria so I didn't have to interact with him."

Her plan didn't work. He was at the court when she arrived. "He was ever so charming. He asked me why I was suing him for maintenance and I told him 'Because I'm struggling you know'." He hadn't paid her anything for two years. Despite his anti-social behavior, he was always able to hold down a reasonable job.

The two of them had a discussion with the woman prosecutor. Shaun told her emphatically that he was not going to pay maintenance because he wanted Ester back. He was told he would have to pay. He still refused, saying, "You can put me in jail. I won't pay a cent."

An embarrassed Ester told the prosecutor, "Leave it, he's making an asshole out of me." As they left the court, he started "charming" her again. His persuasiveness succeeded. "The next thing he had wormed his way back into my life," she said.

"I've got a very soft heart because of my belief. I am with the Christian Motorcyclist's Association Church. It's a happy-clappy type of church."

She was living on an isolated plot at Gerhardsville in Pretoria West, and when she happened to mention that her house had recently been broken into, he insisted on moving back in with her to give her protection. "We talked about getting married again. He told me how he had changed and gave me all kinds of beautiful promises. I foolishly believed him."

Soon after he had moved into her house, he took her for an evening out to a bar in Rosebank to introduce her to some of his friends. She had no way of knowing how drastically a few drinks at a pub were going to change her life.

They were in a jovial mood, drinking away, when one of his friends put his arm on Ester's shoulder. Ludek, who was a "terribly jealous person," started an argument with both of them. They had come in her car and, when she refused to give him the keys, things got very nasty. He knocked her down, and she hit her head on the pavement.

The next thing she remembered was waking up in the bedroom of her home. Looking around, she saw Ludek lying on the floor. He had died as he had lived, violently; shot through the chest. His life had ebbed away in a pool of blood at the age of 30.

Ester did not remember what happened after they left the pub. She had to rely on what relatives told her. "They said my gun and Shaun's were lying on the kitchen table after he was killed. How they got there, I wouldn't know."

"Do you believe Shaun shot himself?" I asked.

"As I've already told you, Shaun often said he was going to commit suicide and I believe he finally did it that night. He shot himself once before, when he was married to another woman for three months after we got divorced. It was a terrible relationship. She was just as mad as he was. He shot himself in the stomach after they had a row about something or other."

Ester was arrested and put in the holding cells at the Erasmia Police Station. The Police did gunpowder tests on her hands and on Shaun's to see if either of them had recently fired a gun. "There was nothing on mine, but his were full of it," she recalled. Bureaucracy being what it is the State still would not drop the murder charge against her. The following morning, she appeared in the Pretoria Magistrate's Court. She pleaded not guilty and was released on bail of R3 000.

Hennie du Plessis, who was employed at one of Armadillo's branches, offered to help Ester when he heard about her arrest. Their Christian belief brought them even closer together. Two years later, they were married with the slur of being a murderess still hanging over her.

"He stood by me through the whole case and everything," she said. "If it wasn't for him, I don't think I would have been here today. Physically, emotionally and mentally he was always with me."

His background was in the secret world of counterintelligence for the apartheid Government. He was captured in Zambia, tried for espionage, and spent five years on death row in that country before being released when the African National Congress came to power in South Africa in 1994.

"Our Government got him out," said Ester. "That was before I met him. A doctor, who went there, certified he had a heart problem, so he was released and deported back to South Africa."

"When the ANC took over they started prosecuting these guys," said George Schurmann, his Pretoria attorney. "We had discussions with the prosecuting authority because they were looking for him. They wanted him to testify against his old mates. But he was never formally charged. In the end they said, "Okay you've paid your dues, so that's it."

"He was a very nice oke, but a dangerous one to get on the wrong side of. It was a long time ago that he was working for the previous Government. Then he gave up that kind of work and started a pastoral service. He went into prisons to help people. So in the end it actually worked out fine."

Both Mariskca and Sane` developed such a close bond with Hennie that they took his surname and called him their father.

An inquest was held into Ludek's death. This dragged on with adjournments for all kinds of trivial reasons. Eventually, seven years after it began, the Magistrate decided there was not sufficient evidence to take the matter any further.

By the time Ester had effectively been found not guilty of murdering Ludek, she was saddled with an even greater burden. It was a life sentence, very different from the kind handed down for murder. For a mother, it was hard to think of anything more heart-rending.

"Just when I thought 'I'm released, my life is coming together now', this thing happened to Mariskca, and it started all over again," she said.

While her mother had to contend with the problems her first husband had brought upon her, Mariskca was showing incredible determination to be treated like any normal child. This was despite needing another much more serious operation in 2000. Because of her gunshot injury she had gradually developed severe scoliosis so, at the age of 12, Dr. Craig operated on her at the Johannesburg Hospital and inserted Harrington rods in her spine to straighten it. There were no complications, and her posture improved.

Mariskca felt she should not have been at the Hope School because the other children were far more disabled than she was. On her own initiative, she applied and was accepted by the Birchleigh Hoerskool. She started there in Grade 8 at the beginning of 2002.

Reporting on Mariskca's abilities when she initially went to Birchleigh, Margaret Thompson, an occupational therapist, stated: "Mariskca was assertive; had her say; was organized; positive; outgoing; self-confident; a leader; took pride in her appearance; was polite and ladylike and took part in every school function. In athletics, she was able to throw the shot and discus, and she also took part in the school play."

Most of these attributes were soon to change after 26 September 2002. That was when her life and that of her mother were drastically altered once again.

During a routine check-up at the Johannesburg Hospital in February 2002, x-rays showed that one of the rods in her spine had broken. By this time, Dr. Craig had left the country, so she was seen by Dr. Richard Kyte. He informed her parents that, as the bones in her spine had fused successfully, in spite of the breakage, the rods should be removed to prevent any future complications.

After that, Mariskca went backwards and forwards to the hospital and was even admitted on one occasion. They kept sending her home because there was no intensive care unit bed available for her to go into immediately after her operation.

Eventually Mariskca was admitted, only to find that Dr. Kyte had been transferred to Baragwanath Hospital, so her case was assigned to Dr. Lieberthal.

It was mystifying that Lieberthal was allowed to even look at patients there when this unlucky little girl crossed his path. He was already being investigated for using what were, literally, the nuts and bolts of his profession that had been purchased from his own company at greatly inflated prices to the Johannesburg General.

As he was not on the staff, but worked there on a sort of charitable basis, there should have been no problem getting rid of him straight away.

Unfortunately, his star quality reputation appears to have made him almost untouchable up to that stage.

Her mother told me he was "so charming" to her daughter when they first met. "He said to her, 'Tell me what else is bothering you? I'm going to make you beautiful'. She complained about part of a rib that was sticking out and he assured her, 'I'm going to remove that for you, as well'. This pleased her. 'That would be wonderful,' she said."

When Lieberthal did the operation, assisted by Dr. Niazi, he removed the rods and inserted screws because he claimed her spine was unstable.

"Dr. Lieberthal told us the operation would not take long, only about an hour," Ester told me. "We got worried when Mariskca had not come back from theatre two hours later. We asked one of the nurses what was happening and we were told everything was going well."

Mariskca was in theatre for nearly six hours and then moved to ICU. The frightened child came round feverish, vomiting, and in severe pain. Then she stopped breathing. It was only through the quick intervention of the nursing staff that she was resuscitated.

"She complained to my husband that she was very sore on her one side," Ester continued, "so he and a nurse helped to turn her and there was a lot of blood under her. She told her father that she could not feel her legs, and she cried a lot. She kept asking Hennie to promise that she would not be paralyzed."

Dr. Niazi was called, and he immediately realized there was a problem, but neither he nor the sisters could get hold of Lieberthal. "I also tried to contact him without success," the girl's mother said. "Shortly afterwards, we saw the story in The Star about Dr. Lieberthal, so you can imagine how worried we were then, especially as Dr. Niazi said he could not tell us what had gone wrong as he was only the assistant."

Mariskca was moved into an ordinary ward with her anxious mother by her side, but her condition did not improve. In desperation, Ester left a message on Lieberthal's cell phone, asking him to contact her. She spent the night beside her daughter's bed wrestling with this terrible Lieberthal nightmare.

"When I woke up that morning, Dr. Lieberthal was standing at the end of the bed. I obviously expected him to tell me what was wrong with Mariskca, but he just walked out without saying anything and disappeared. I phoned him again on his cell phone, but he did not speak to me, so I left a message urging him to explain what had gone wrong."

He was toying with their emotions, playing a cruel cat-and-mouse game.

Much like Ester's former husband, who could not face up to the fact that he had shot his baby daughter, Lieberthal was in denial about the reality of what he had done to the same girl.

The elusive a surgeon sent Ester an SMS saying he would go and see Mariskca that afternoon at four o'clock. She and her husband were there waiting for him when he finally arrived in the ward.

"He said that the problem was caused by swelling," Ester said. "He blamed other people who had worked with him for what had happened. The anesthetist, he claimed, had caused Mariskca to stop breathing. He refused to admit he had made a terrible mistake.

"When he operated, he didn't touch the rib, thank goodness. Otherwise, she would have had no ribs left, probably."

Describing the situation briefly in the hospital 20 days after the operation, Dr. Niazi wrote, "Post-operative complication was complete paraplegia. Dr. Lieberthal was informed many times by myself, family, and ICU telephonically, but was not available."

After Mariskca's stepfather had complained to Sagie Pillay, the hospital manager, Mariskca was shuffled backwards and forwards by car to other hospitals because there was no ambulance available. She was sent for scans, but they did not show what had actually happened. A myelogram was also tried, yet this too was unsuccessful.

"At the meeting we had at the hospital, we were told they were sorry Mariskca was paralyzed, but that we would just have to carry on with our lives," Ester told me.

Giving his opinion in a medico-legal report completed for Mariskca's legal action that followed, Dr. Herman Edeling, a neurosurgeon, stated that no consent was obtained for the insertion of screws or any other form of spinal instrumentation. The consent form had evidently meant nothing to Lieberthal because it only authorized the "removal of instrumentation, spine."

He was particularly harsh on Lieberthal. "Six days after the operation, Dr. Lieberthal appears to have written a note in the bed letter (letter of medical necessity) for the first time. He recorded her sensory level to be at L2, whereas the nursing records and the history provided by the patient indicated a higher sensory level. In his opinion, the screws were in a satisfactory position, which is contradicted by the post-operative x-rays. He suggested the administration of Decadron (cortisone used to reduce inflammation), which would have been of no benefit. He failed to advise any treatment which may have helped to reduce the neurological damage."

Mariskca went home in a wheelchair with no feeling in her legs from the waist down. Her worst fears had become a reality. Unknown to her, the Butcher of Rosebank had lived up to his terrifying reputation.

Realizing that Mariskca and her parents still did not know the exact extent of what had happened to her, one of the teachers at her school put them in touch with radiologist Dr. Wim Burger at the Arwyp Medical Centre nearby. The scan he did on Mariskca, free of charge, showed what the staff at the government hospitals had been unable to see, and that was that the screws had gone into the spinal cord.

Dr. Burger told Ester to take her daughter back to the Johannesburg General to have the screws removed immediately. There she was seen by the new professor of orthopedics, Professor Lukhele.

Ester described him as "excellent." Mariskca really trusted him because he understood how she felt. He promised her he would remove the screws himself and not let anybody else touch her. He booked her in that same night and took the screws out the following morning. "I'm not sure if it was him or somebody at Dr. Burger's who said if they had removed the screws within a few days she might still have got back to what she was before, but they left it too late. I sent Dr. Lieberthal an SMS saying, 'May God forgive you'. My husband wanted to kill him."

In another medical-legal report, neurosurgeon Dr. Gian Marus described exactly what had happened and who was to blame. "The usual cause of immediate post-operative paralysis relates to direct spinal cord injury. The cause of the spinal cord injury is clearly identified by the CT scan done on 6/11/2002. These scans show the right sided screws at L1 and L2 penetrated into the spinal canal and their course would be expected to transect the spinal cord–conus and cauda equina. This would be regarded as negligence and from the hospital records Dr. Lieberthal is clearly identified as the surgeon involved in the procedure."

Attempting to justify his client's actions, Lieberthal's attorney, Krawitz, wrote that Lieberthal had been "one of a team of doctors" who operated on Mariskca. "New instruments were placed in the spine nowhere near the level of paralysis she is now suffering. She was paralyzed at vertebra L1, whereas the instrumentation was inserted at L3, L4, T7 and T8."

When Mariskca was able to return to school, a welcome party was organized for her. The school did its best to make life as easy as possible for her and 16-year-old Riaan Louw helped her up and down the steps in her wheelchair between classes. It was hardly surprising that she was often tearful and depressed.

She was now dependent on her mother as never before. Lieberthal had completely ruined another life.

Mrs. du Plessis could not hide the bitterness that came through when she talked about her daughter's mental reaction to what had happened "Mariskca felt in her heart; how can he live with himself knowing that he's done these things to these people and he just carries on as if there is nothing wrong? She thinks that Lieberthal gets a kick out of making people the way that he did. You know, with us being Christians it's very important that when you've done something wrong you must admit it, repent and ask for forgiveness, you know, which he didn't do."

Two years after Mariskca was paralyzed she sent a pitiful letter to Lieberthal. "Wynne, people say forgive and forget," it began. "I have forgiven you, but how can I forget if my whole life is full of memories and struggle?"

She was particularly concerned that here was a man who could never apologies for what he had done. "You looked like such a trustworthy and loyal person. Why do you hide when you've done something wrong? Why can't you just say you're sorry when you've messed up?"

It was clear that it would have meant a great deal to her if he had just been big enough to admit he was wrong. If only she had been able to revive the compassion he had shown when he broke down in tears in front of that other girl when he was a much younger doctor. Cold as the scalpel he used to take Mariskca's life away, he did not reply.

When I saw her and her mother, Mariskca had left school and was working in a call center. Her life would forever be a constant reminder of the surgeon who had let her down so badly in more ways than one.

Her troubled life was made even more tragic because her stepfather, to whom she had become much attached, was no longer there. As if she and her mother had not had enough heart-rending experiences to contend with, he was killed on Valentine's Day a year before my visit to the family. He was riding his motorbike from work when a pickup truck crashed into him as he was crossing at some traffic lights. The driver didn't even have a license.

Mariskca's plight was cushioned to some degree when her claim against the Gauteng Province, as owners of the Johannesburg Hospital, was finalized early in 2005 after the Premier, in his capacity as head of the Province, admitted negligence.

There's nothing like a big payout for attracting the investment gurus. The newspaper story about Mariskca newly acquired fortune had them knocking on the door of the family home.

A representative from Deloitte and Touche, the multinational accounting and financial advisory firm, were the first to arrive. "They wanted to tell me how to invest the money," Ester pointed out. "They went on what they saw in the paper. For some reason, our lawyer didn't want me to tell the reporter that he took 25 percent. They thought I had R6-million, but we only got R4-million in the end. I don't think this was enough money for them, so they referred me to somebody else. When the second guy came I said to him, 'Let me be quite honest with you I don't trust investment people because there's plenty old people who were robbed of their pensions. I'm going to invest the money myself'.

"So I put it in a money market account, where it's safe, because there were a lot of things I had to do with it. I mean, if I can't make her life easier with the money that she's got, what does it mean? It means nothing."

Chapter 15

Doctors Eat Doctor

Surely a collection of complaints compiled by three prominent orthopedic surgeons, involving back operations done on 32 patients by Lieberthal should have been given top priority by the Health Professions Council when it was submitted in 2000? This was especially so since one of the people on the list had died under suspicious circumstances.

In May 2004, the Council's President, Professor Nicky Padayachee, made a startling admission to the Sunday Times. "Our first responsibility is to protect people. Instead, there had been a tendency to focus on the interests of professional members." Was this why the complaint from the three specialists was perhaps dropped into a "dead" file?

My guess was that, in the entire history of the Health Professions Council, it had never had a list of complaints of this magnitude compiled by doctors against another doctor. It should have sent alarm bells ringing through every corner of the HPCSA. These, however, remained depressingly silent until they were jingled into action by the media publicity that Lieberthal finally got for his awful deeds, two years after the three doctors submitted their grievances.

The Registrar, Advocate Boyce Mkhize, gave me this inexplicable explanation for this monumental blunder. In the metamorphosis of his Council, reconstituted after 1994 when a democratically elected government came to power, they did not have a coordinating system. If several complaints were lodged against a particular doctor, the Council would not necessarily have been aware that the same practitioner was involved in each instance.

It was a deplorable excuse that was hardly a valid reason for shelving a case that the trio of specialists had already consolidated into a long list of people, who Lieberthal had operated on from as far back as December 1996, when he started orthopedics on his own.

"Even if there was no consolidation, 32 cases from three doctors in itself should have been dealt with more promptly, shouldn't it?" I said to Mkhize, watching him intently to see how he would react. "My impression is that it was an unwritten code in the medical profession that doctors did not report doctors, especially on such a large scale. And that was what should have made this case even more worthy of prompt action."

"Most definitely, most definitely," was his hard-to-believe reply in view of what had actually happened. "Once the issue came to light, and we saw the gravity of the complaints, we then put measures in place to expedite them. Hence the swift inspection we conducted at his practice. All the processes were basically fast tracked because it dawned on us that this was a little bit more serious than perhaps we may have anticipated."

The complaints from the surgeons showed conclusively that "fast tracking" was not one of the Council's attributes, especially when it came to its favorite spinal surgeon. The letter addressed to the Chairman of the HPCSA was dated 31 October 2000 and had the names of the following orthopedic surgeons at the bottom: Dr. James Craig, Dr. Anthony Thomas, and Dr. Jos van Niekerk.

The document gave the impression that they were such reluctant complainants that it took them four years to pluck up the courage to take the final step towards officially accusing a colleague of a huge inventory of serious botch-ups. Having done this, they must have been disappointed by the length of time the Council took to react. Yet none of them, it appears, made any inquiries as to the progress of their complaint as it gathered dust in some seldom visited cabinet. Had the media not exposed Lieberthal, the indications were that their efforts could still be languishing in the archives of the HPCSA to this day.

Van Niekerk was the only one of the three who was prepared to discuss their letter with me at a stage when it had already been made public at an HPCSA hearing. The other two behaved like undercover agents whose activities had to remain a secret in the interests of the state.

Craig was by then working for the National Health Service in England. He did not answer several emails I sent him. Thomas, too, was just as publicity shy. When I asked if I could come and see him about the letter at the Morningside Clinic where both he and Van Niekerk practiced, he said, "Well the trouble is, that's confidential."

"It's not confidential because it's now public knowledge," I replied forcefully.

"Well, the letter we would have sent is confidential to the HPCSA. I would have to speak to our Orthopaedic Association to find out what the ethics are." He undertook to come back to me, but he never did.

Van Niekerk, on the other-hand, was commendably cooperative when I saw him in his rooms in May 2007. Certificates on the wall recorded his prestigious past. One was when he was made an International Member of the American Orthopedic Foot and Ankle Society in 1997. Another showed that he had been President of the South African Orthopaedic Association from 1993 to 1995, and subsequently became a life member.

I asked him to tell me briefly what the problems were regarding the people on the list. “A variety of things,” he said. “Dr. Craig collected the majority of them because his practice was confined to spinal surgery. They were people with bad results, multiple operations, and things like that. I’m not a spinal surgeon by any manner of means.” His specialty was feet and ankles.

“Did the Medical Council acknowledge receiving your complaint?” I asked.

“I’m just trying to think who in the end really dispatched it. I think the short answer is probably no. They received it obviously because that’s been proved. I can’t recall receiving or being told we got an acknowledgement that they’ve got it.”

Intrigued to know what they did during the period when their report was “lost,” I asked, “During those two years did you people, at any stage, say, ‘Hey, what’s happening about this?’”

“The way the Medical Council functions is that a complaint goes to them. They then write to the doctor and that can go on for quite a long time. We thought we’ve done our bit.”

Amazed by their passivity, I said, “You were waiting for them …”

“To come up with something. We’ve put the file on their desk and we trusted they would get on with it. Now how they would have chosen to do it is obviously their right.”

A learned-looking man, whose retirement was not far off, he said that sometimes the patients listed, wanted a second opinion after being treated by Lieberthal. He saw one or two through the work he did for the Government’s Compensation Commissioner. People who were injured at work could make a claim and they would be assessed as being X percent disabled. If they were not happy with this, they could appeal. That was when specialists like him were called in to give an independent opinion.

Paying tribute to them, I said, “I must commend the three of you because, in my limited experience, doctors don’t stick their necks out on things like this.”

“Well, sometimes you think you should.”

“Is it fair to say it is extremely unusual for doctors to complain to the Medical Council about other doctors?”

“It’s definitely not commonly done, no.”

“We the undersigned”, the letter began, “after extensive deliberation approach you and state that, in our opinion, the practice of Dr. Lieberthal falls far short of the standard acceptable for a qualified orthopedic surgeon, even more so taking into consideration that he professes to have a special interest in spinal surgery. The areas are as follows:

1. Indications for surgery.

We contend that in a number of cases the indications for surgery either were totally absent or were of a very flimsy nature. By this we mean that no pathology had been demonstrated before surgery by any investigations or that the pathology was grossly misrepresented and furthermore that a reasonable period of conservative treatment had never been offered to the patient.

2. Multiple surgery

There are a number of cases where multiple surgery, i.e. an operation to the cervical and the lumbar (in other words top and bottom) spine were performed on the same patient under the same anesthetic. This type of procedure is not an internationally recognized surgical practice and we can find no motivation or reason why this would be of benefit to the patient. In many of the cases, the converse is true.

3. Drug prescription

A number of cases are recorded where exceedingly high doses of potentially habit-forming drugs had been prescribed for patients for extended periods of time without the necessary medical supervision.

4. Other problems

On assessing matters that have come to our attention we note what appears to be, in our opinion, exceptionally high levels of the following complications:

i) Wrong level surgery.

ii) Nerve root damage.

iii) Dural tears and leaks.

iv) Post-operative sepsis.

"We respectively request the above matters to be investigated by yourselves. We wish to stress that we have been considering the matter for a long time and now feel forced, by circumstances, to act. This will be borne out if note is taken of the period over which these matters have been collected by the doctors involved."

It had been four years from when the first person on the list that followed had been operated on by Lieberthal.

The final sentence was a tactful hint that the HPCSA should hurry up and investigate this matter. "We are also led to believe that Dr. Lieberthal may be considering emigrating to Australia." That, of course, was where his second oldest brother, Isidore, had started his own textile business years earlier.

Attached to the letter was a list of all the patients and documents to support the allegations. Among those I have spotlighted are:

Freda Polak. 12/12/1996. She had a fusion and screw fixation done on her by Lieberthal because of a nerve root injury, but when Craig saw her eight days before her operation, he could find no signs of nerve root damage, judging by her clinical records.

Aubrey Miller. 02/07/1997. Before his operation there was evidence of narrowing of the central spinal canal at two levels and a disc protrusion at another part of the spine. He was treated by inserting cages with a pedicle screw fixation only at the level where there was a disc protrusion.

Carla du Toit. 21/07/1997. She had a titanium cage and other hardware inserted in her back in the area of a fractured vertebra. But a screw was put into the disc space between the vertebrae instead of into the bone itself.

Gredna Bush. 12/08/1997. She consulted Craig in August 1997 and he saw no indication that she needed further back surgery. One month later, Lieberthal extended her spine fusion, and the operation was complicated by a spinal fluid leak. Then, in April 1999, Lieberthal did another operation to revise the instrumentation that had previously been inserted. Afterwards, she had severe left sciatica and back pain. When Craig saw her in February 2000, she seemed dependent on various pain-killing drugs.

Robin Gordon. 26/08/1997. He had two spine operations a month apart when the second one was not indicated.

Malgorzata Pilsniak. 23/10/1997. Regarding her operation it stated, "Cages technically not well performed, i.e. they are not parallel in the disc space and they have been associated with a worsening of the right sciatica symptoms following surgery".

Joel Michael Rothbart. 13/11/1997. "Indications for the 5th lower back operation are not well defined, and it had been the opinion of neurosurgeons Dr. C. van Heerden and Dr. I. Weinberg and two other senior doctors at Johannesburg Hospital that the patient did not require surgery."

Elise Kleynhans. 21/11997. She suffered from scoliosis, and Lieberthal did an operation to straighten her spine. "But her deformity has increased following surgery," the letter stated.

Gregory Jarvis. 30/03/1998. He was only aged 19 when he was advised by Lieberthal to have a back operation, which would have included a fusion. This did not seem indicated according to Craig, who saw him for a second opinion.

Mr. Z. Zwane. 23/04/1998. Lieberthal went to Ladysmith to treat him when three of his vertebrae were fractured. But one of them was not included by the instrumentation that was inserted.

Harry Higgs. 13/05/1999. He had three neck operations in which a graft was displaced, resulting in swallowing and breathing difficulties after the second operation. This 30-year-old patient was given a letter within three months of the last operation stipulating that he should be pensioned off by his employer on medical grounds, when not enough time had been allowed for normal convalescence.

Ernest Waczkow. 18/05/1999. This 18-year-old underwent a laminectomy, as well as fusions with pedicle screw fixation that was complicated by an infection in the wound.

Rene Papadopoulos. 10/06/1999. Lieberthal advised her to have neck surgery, but in the opinion of both Craig and Van Heerden she did not need this.

Edward Perlman. 17/08/1999. At the age of 69, he was given a lumbar spine fusion. But the instrumentation that was inserted resulted in him having a flat back deformity. "This is a technically poor result of a pedicle screw fixation method," the letter lamented.

Everest Ferreira. 20/05/2000. He had five operations. The instrumentation had to be redone twice after the first operation and, after the fourth one, he developed a deep wound infection which required surgical treatment.

Johanna Sharp, Constance Heywood, and Juanita Hobson all developed wound infections after their operations in 2000. Lieberthal opened Sharp's back on five occasions.

Brian Flynn. 14/07/2000. He had neck and lumbar spine surgery under the same anesthetic. This was complicated by the temporary loss of his voice and difficulty in swallowing. The plate that was put in his neck was poorly applied and disc degeneration at one particular level was not addressed. Following surgery, he had to be re-admitted to hospital and put into the Intensive Care Unit because he developed pneumonia and septicemia. The final blow for Flynn was that "this surgery and its complications resulted in the patient losing the opportunity to take up a teaching post in the United Kingdom".

The most controversial of the 32 involved Maureen Gainsford. She was aged 61 when she went to see Dr. Andrezej (known as Andrew) Dybala at the Kensington Clinic, not far from her home. Dybala was a Polish orthopedic surgeon who had trained with Lieberthal at Wits University. Backs apparently were not his forte, so he passed these cases on to his old classmate. He appears to have continued doing this long after he must have heard on the medical grapevine that the glittering star he had known at university had lost his shine completely. When I asked him if he had been "happy" with the treatment his patients received after he had sent them to Lieberthal he said, "Yes, generally, yes."

Gainsford was suffering from acute sciatica when Lieberthal admitted her to the Linksfield Park Clinic. There he operated on her lower back; removed what he described as a "large cyst" and did a fusion in January 1997.

Gainsford died two days after her operation. This raised the question: Was her death caused by any negligence that could be attributed to Lieberthal?

"I went with my wife to see Lieberthal," her husband Neville told me. He had since remarried and was living in Durban. "He told her, 'It's a piece of cake. No problem, we'll have you walking within a week with no pains or anything'. He was quite convincing."

His experience was just as disturbing as those other people had, when they tried to get in touch with Lieberthal after an operation. "We could never speak to him. He just seemed to disappear off the scene." While the operation was going on, Gainsford became concerned that it was taking longer than he had expected. So he spoke to a sister. "'Don't worry,' she told me, 'nothing is going wrong'." After the operation, his wife had to be put on life support because she couldn't breathe. She soon recovered and was taken to the ward. "She told me they would be getting her up the following morning," her husband said.

He had taken a few days off work to be with his wife in hospital and, now that she was improving, he went back to the factory where he was a production manager. "Then they phoned me from the hospital to tell me I must come quickly." With a tremor in his voice, he added, "I got there too late. She was dead." He had been married for 37 years, and the couple had three sons, who were all grown up when their mother died.

The Johannesburg Inquest Magistrate, Scholtz Maritz, now had the job of determining whether anybody could be held accountable for Gainsford's death. He conducted his inquiry in an extremely thorough fashion by exploring all possible causes.

He obtained reports from Dr. Patricia Klepp, the state pathologist who performed the post-mortem; Professor Charles Isaacson, from the Department of Pathology at the Wits Medical School; as well as Dr. Craig. There was also a letter from Lieberthal replying to Isaacson's report, as well as other documents in the file.

According to Isaacson, on the second or third day after the operation Gainsford went to the toilet by herself and when she returned to her bed, she had a seizure and died soon afterwards. "The embolus is the blood clot," he wrote, "which traveled in the bloodstream to both lungs and was the final cause of death. It would probably have originated in the calves of the legs." He referred to a "pin" Lieberthal had inserted in the woman's spine. It had protruded into the abdominal cavity where it caused bleeding. He suggested that an orthopedic expert should be consulted to decide whether the site of the pin and "the resultant hemorrhage in the surrounding tissue, constituted medical negligence or not." It was at this point that Dr. Craig was asked for his opinion.

In his defense, Lieberthal said that the "pin" was in fact a screw and only a cold-hearted person like him could have described the way it was inserted as "entirely correct." The bleeding that resulted from the screw penetrating the abdominal cavity was "insignificant," and unrelated to her pulmonary embolism, he claimed. In keeping with his long record of refusing to admit he had made a mistake, his letter ended, "The procedure was uneventful and according to my opinion well performed."

That might have been his biased belief, but it was certainly not the conclusion that Dr. Craig came to. "The site of the pin and the resultant hemorrhage in the surrounding tissue does indeed constitute negligence. But it is not possible to make a direct link between the pedicle screw, which penetrated the anterior cortex of the L4 vertebral body, and the thrombosis in the deep calf veins."

Isaacson also felt that Lieberthal could not be held responsible for the woman's death. "It should be accentuated that, even if the operation procedure was done in a negligent manner, the death of the patient was due to pulmonary embolus. This is an accepted complication of any major surgical procedure, although early mobilization of patients after an operation has reduced this complication considerably. Nevertheless, the coagulability of the blood increases immediately after trauma, and during, and for approximately two weeks after, surgery. This explains why deep vein thrombosis often starts during, or shortly after, surgical operations and often extends rapidly to major veins during this period."

Lieberthal was not in the clear yet.

The Magistrate sent a letter to Dr. Klepp stating, "You have suggested that an open inquest be convened to determine whether there was negligence on the part of the treating doctors. The relatives of the deceased are anxious that an open inquest be held."

In South Africa, magistrates usually finalize inquests purely on written evidence. They have the power, where they consider the case warrants it, to order that an inquest be held in open court. It is a more laborious procedure because the witnesses, who are entitled to have legal representation, give oral evidence and can be cross-examined. However, this is seldom done.

"The relatives," Maritz's letter to Klepp continued, "believe that a link can be established between the hemorrhage and the pulmonary embolus. You concluded that the causes of death were two-fold, to wit, 'Intra-abdominal hemorrhage and pulmonary embolism'. This leads me to ask, could the intra-abdominal hemorrhage independently have caused death and can the intra-abdominal hemorrhage be regarded as introductory to the final cause of death? Thirdly, could the intra-abdominal hemorrhage have created a climate conducive to the formation of the deep vein thrombi? Only negligence in the form of an act 'or commission, which brought about death', would allow an open inquest to be convened."

Dr. Klepp, however, doubted if an open inquest would be viable because the post-mortem examination did not show that the screw damage resulted in her death. Anybody could get deep vein thrombosis with embolisation. The person did not need to bleed elsewhere to get it.

Neville Gainsford, who worked for Lasher Tools before he took early retirement and then got another job at a smaller firm, told me that he and his sons spoke to the Magistrate. "We wanted to know if we should sue. The screw that Dr. Lieberthal stuck in her spine was sticking out 18 millimeters too much. But the Magistrate told us that there was no definite proof that his negligence cause her death and, as doctors all belonged to the same 'club', he didn't think it was worth us pursuing it any further. It was a big blow to us all, and my sons took it particularly badly."

Two years after Gainsford died, the Magistrates ruled that nobody could be held responsible for her death.

Once again, Lieberthal had narrowly escaped having to appear in a criminal court. He was free to carry on operating on his unsuspecting patients.

When it came to mudslinging, Lieberthal could do it with the best of them.

He produced plenty of it through his advocate against the three specialists in his reply to the HPCSA.

Advocate David Goldblum's letter, written in long-winded legalese, was dated 28 August 2001, ten months after the date on the complaint. It consisted of the following: explanations, vilification of his accusers, and threats.

Within one month of Lieberthal commencing practice in 1996, Craig told Dr. Lieberthal that he had received complaints that he was not keeping colleagues informed of the "on goings" in his practice. A month after that, Lieberthal was again "summonsed" to see Craig, who accused him of not charging his patients appropriately. Lieberthal explained that he had got the rates from Dr. Nainkin. Since then, he had been charging the tariffs Craig had given him.

Lieberthal was particularly "shocked" by the allegations being made against him because, while he was a surgeon in training, Craig was always available to assist him academically and technically. "This changed completely when my client went into practice, and, in fact, started building a successful practice, which is clearly indicative of professional jealousy. My client can only assume that Dr. Craig's nose was put out of joint due to the tremendous success and following which my client attained in a short period of time." Craig had made "seriously defamatory allegations to certain lay people in the hospital industry" against Lieberthal which had "injured his good name and reputation".

"It is interesting to note," Goldblum continued, "that Dr. Craig fails to mention previous failed surgeries by other orthopedic colleagues who operated on my client's patients prior to him. It appears that Dr. Craig has embarked on a personal vendetta against my client attempting to discredit him and destroy his good name and practice."

According to Lieberthal, several newly qualified orthopedic surgeons had some kind of problem with Van Niekerk because he had made "many defamatory" allegations against his colleagues, including Lieberthal. "In this regard, the necessary actions are being instituted." This could not have been true because, nearly six years later, when I interviewed Van Niekerk, no action had been taken against him.

Goldblum maintained his client operated on "Thursday and Friday" at provincial hospitals doing adult and pediatric spinal cases at no charge. This was another fabrication, unless Lieberthal had an uncanny ability to be in two places at once. Alternatively, if it were true, then a court was misled when Lieberthal claimed that, from 1996 to February 2003, he made use of the theatre at the Rosebank Clinic for "the entire day on Tuesdays and Thursdays".

The submission that Lieberthal had been asked by Professor George to plan the new curriculum at Wits University "for the teaching program for medical students as it pertains to the spine" was also misleading. George told me he asked Lieberthal to do this around 2001 or 2002, "But he was too busy,

I think, in his private practice." Lieberthal never did unnecessary operations, Goldblum continued. He only operated "after all avenues of conservative treatment had been exhausted" and if the "indications for surgery were supported by clinical evaluation and radiological evidence". The patient was "always told of any risks or possible complications prior to surgery".

The fact that numerous orthopedic surgeons referred cases to his client showed that Lieberthal had an "impeccable standing amongst most of his orthopedic colleagues". If this were so, why was it that the only name that I came across was that of Dr. Dybala? Also, why didn't Lieberthal name them, to enable the HPSC to get references from them?

His advocate countered the criticism that it was wrong for Lieberthal to perform multiple surgeries under the same anesthetic by referring to an article in Campbell's Orthopedics, which endorsed his client's single procedure and refuted Craig's claim that this was not internationally recognized. In 1995 at the South African Orthopedic Association's Congress in Durban, Lieberthal presented an original paper about multiple surgeries at the same sitting. "And my client was personally informed of the benefits of this surgical procedure by Dr. Craig himself." The article was published in the South African Bone and Joint Journal and was elected as the best paper at the Congress.

The allegation that Lieberthal prescribed Schedule 7 drugs unnecessarily was unfounded because he only did this after he had "exhausted all conservative avenues". It was only in the event of "persisting grade four pain" that he prescribe Schedule 6 medication, such as Pethidine.

"In none of the alleged cases did my client cause nerve root damage. And as regards dural tears and leaks, every surgeon, including my client, will have patients who present with these problems, after surgical procedures. This is a common complication and after each surgical procedure the risk of these increases. Dr. Craig has himself had these problems, which he documented in the South African Journal of Bone and Joint Surgery. The risk of infection is especially prevalent in cases of revision surgery and medically compromised patients," Goldblum conceded. However, Craig had got it wrong in the cases that he referred to, as tests showed there was no sepsis.

Goldblum threatened to take whatever legal action he considered appropriate over the claim that his client was emigrating to Australia. This was not true. And it was "clearly defamatory as patients would not consult him if they were led to believe that he intended emigrating".

He also complained that it appeared that Doctors Thomas and Van Niekerk had simply endorsed Craig's allegations without actually examining any of the patients themselves.

Completing his portrait of the perfect doctor, Goldblum went on, "My client gave all his patients the option—especially those who expressed anxiety about any surgical procedures—of obtaining a second opinion and, in this regard, he always furnished three alternative orthopedic surgeons, being Dr. Nainkin, Dr. Meerkotter, and Dr. Craig. These surgeons' names were listed on the x-ray packets, together with their telephone numbers". Why did I never come across any evidence to support this? And, if he was at loggerheads with Craig, is it likely that he would have recommended him?

Goldblum put the complaints from the three doctors down to "professional jealousy" because "there was no foundation whatsoever" for them. He warned that "every available legal avenue will be utilized in order to refute all the allegations. This will include, should it be necessary, an application to the High Court together with an action in the Constitutional Court for discrimination, as this is a human rights violation."

Now that the allegations from the three prominent orthopedic surgeons had surfaced, would they be enough to get Lieberthal into the dock at a full Medical Council disciplinary hearing? Or would his explanations be accepted once again?

Chapter 16

Scalpels Are Out

If Lieberthal was squirming under the barrage of publicity he was getting, what hit him next was an even heavier blow to his perceived image of the brilliant surgeon whose work was nothing short of infallible. It came just four months after his name had become synonymous with bungled back operations.

Could the smooth charmer talk his way out of this one?

In February 2003, Lieberthal got a hand-delivered letter from Richard Treisman, the Legal Advisor of the Netcare Group, owners of the Rosebank Clinic, as well as the premises opposite the hospital where Lieberthal had his rooms. The spine surgeon had become a leper, too infectious to be allowed to remain in his own hospital.

His record of bringing hundreds of patients to the hospital over the years was not going to be enough to earn him a reprieve. Like so many of his patients, he was about to be discharged as an extremely angry and unhappy person, without so much as an Aspirin to dull the pain.

"It is with regret that we must inform you," the forbidding type began, "that a decision has been taken by Management at the Hospital and endorsed by the Board of Directors of Network Healthcare Holdings Limited (known as Netcare), to terminate you're admitting rights to the Hospital with immediate effect."

Treisman told Lieberthal that it was "common cause" that he had made statements, both written and oral, "that you hold the Hospital and its staff responsible for conspiring against you and being responsible for the unfortunate situation in which you find yourself. You have in fact gone as far as to request compensation from the Hospital".

It must have been abundantly clear to Lieberthal that his sell-by-date had finally arrived. In case he did not get the message the letter added: "The relationship that exists between yourself, the Hospital and the staff, has reached a level which is inconsistent with an ongoing working relationship and in the circumstances it cannot endure. You will be allowed to complete treating your patients currently under your supervision in the Hospital, but will not be permitted to continue using the Hospital's operating facilities."

Confiscating Lieberthal's theatre time could be a death blow to his practice. Hospitals did their best to attract specialists, so a money spinner like Lieberthal might still be able to resurrect his career elsewhere. By 1 June 2003, he also had to vacate his rooms, which he occupied on a monthly tenancy, on the same floor as the Centre of Sports Medicine in Sturdee House, Rosebank.

Krawitz, Lieberthal's attorney, replied saying Treisman's letter was an "unlawful repudiation of the agreement between yourself and our client". Lieberthal accepted this, but reserved his right to sue. "We hereby notify you that our client intends instituting action against you for damages."

His client had suffered further damages because now no other hospital in South Africa was prepared to provide him with "admission rights". It looked as though Lieberthal's big mouth and aggressive approach had cut his main artery completely this time. However, the indestructible doctor was showing no signs of succumbing.

Krawitz also took Netcare's employees to task for "defamatory remarks" about his client. He warned that "unless you take the necessary steps to restrain them our client will have no alternative but to approach the media to safeguard his rights and to present his side of the story".

Considering that this doctor had done nothing but castigate the media, this comical idea showed how disturbed his thinking was.

Lieberthal was not going to let the massive Netcare Group, which made a R659-million profit and had numerous hospitals under its jurisdiction in 2003, push him around, especially as he believed that right was on his side. Towards the end of that year, Lieberthal began an action for damages against it in the High Court in Johannesburg. It evidently did not concern him that his cases against The Star and Primedia had not yet been finalized.

To begin with, Lieberthal demanded R5-million for loss of earnings for being ejected from the Clinic and a further R10-million for defamation. In his summons he blamed the Matron Joan Shewan as well as Sisters Dirkie Theunissen, Trudy Swart, Rosemary Clarke, Karen Botha and a sixth person he named only as Sister Priscilla, for defaming him. Botha was not in fact a nurse; she was the secretary of the orthopedic ward.

He alleged that what the Matron and the Sisters told patients would have been understood to mean that he was "not a reputable orthopedic surgeon; was not a properly qualified doctor; paralyzed many of his patients due to negligence or other unlawful conduct; ruined people's lives; did not follow the Hippocratic Oath; was a dishonorable, untrustworthy individual, and caused death or anguish to his patients instead of giving them the necessary medical assistance." By immortalizing these highly charged, exaggerated words in the court records, he was certainly not improving his image.

Lieberthal was determined to do a lot more than ruffle feathers among the nightingales. They would regret maligned him, even if Netcare, their employer, was not taking him seriously. In May 2003, just before he began his action for damages against Netcare, he lodged a "formal complaint" with the Nursing Council of South Africa in Pretoria against these soft targets. He was clearly aiming to have the nurses amputated from their profession. Presumably, he thought that, if the Nursing Council was to side with him, this would strengthen his case against Netcare.

The loyalty that nurses had for him that Sister Vos had talked about had evidently become decidedly anemic since her days in theatre. Having retired by the time the hemorrhaging began in earnest, she had no firsthand knowledge of how bad things had become.

He complained that in the early part of 2002 the old nursing staff in the orthopedic section was replaced by new members. Of these he singled out Sisters Theunissen, Clarke and Swart as the main culprits. "I became aware of an undercurrent of insubordination in this particular ward pertaining to unprofessional conduct in that these sisters actively canvassed my patients to see another doctor." That must have been the sin of all sins among the subservient nursing staff. Had they forgotten the number one nursing commandment: Thou shalt never ever doubt the sublime ability of thy Gods, the doctors, or speak ill of them. He castigated all three of them for not carrying out routine instructions.

To support his allegations, he sent a wad of statements. They were described as "affidavits" but most of them were not in the proper legal form having not been sworn to in front of a Commissioner of Oaths. The majority were poorly written by hand with the same phrases repeated in different statements. Then too, as my inquiries revealed, some of them were extremely suspect. It looked as though many of his hand-picked witnesses would have been hard pressed to justify their claims, had they been forced to appear at any type of inquiry where they would have been subjected to cross-examination.

The majority of the statements were no holds barred, vicious attempts to blacken the names of the nurses as well as Dr. Brad Hoffmann, who Lieberthal seemed to regard as his most bitter rival. As Lieberthal had demonstrated before, with his court actions, this academically brilliant man was the class dunce when it came to recognizing that the poison he was spreading to get revenge was having a boomerang effect on his own reputation.

Maria Rapoo, a sister at the Rosebank Clinic, who had worked there for three years, was supposed to have signed her statement on Christmas Eve in 2002.In it she claimed that she heard Theunissen telling Matron Shewan that Lieberthal was "not a good surgeon and that he kills and paralyses his patients". She claimed she had also heard these two and Sister Swart saying that Dr. Lieberthal should not be operating on patients and all of them should be told to use Dr. Hoffmann. Sisters Theunissen and Swart and the Matron had a vendetta against Lieberthal and were "hell bent on destroying him".

Sister Theunissen was continually touting for Dr. Hoffmann. In the case of Samantha Mashanini, she heard Sister Theunissen telling student nurse Johanna Kganyago to go and tell Samantha's mother that Lieberthal had "messed her daughter up" and that they should go and see Dr. Hoffmann.

Rapoo added that Sister Swart had influenced a Mrs. Musgrove to go to Dr. Hoffmann and had said, "Dr. Hoffmann does not have any patients. Those that he does have are those that were stolen from Dr. Lieberthal. Since Dr. Lieberthal has not been operating at the Rosebank Clinic, the ground floor ward had fallen to pieces as there are no patients being admitted, except for small cases from Dr. Ferguson and minor blocks done by Dr. Hoffmann."

This statement was not in proper affidavit form but another one she signed eight months later appeared to be done correctly. It had evidently been submitted as part of the nurses" defense and was an almost complete denial of what was in the document that Lieberthal had produced to the Nursing Council.

Rapoo's was now saying that the first statement had been altered without her knowledge. On several occasions she overheard Theunissen suggesting to patients that they should get a second opinion because "Dr. Lieberthal's patients were deteriorating in the ward and she was concerned about their wellbeing". She had never worked with Sister Swart and had not heard Matron Shewan telling Lieberthal's patients to consult Dr. Hoffmann.

Mildred Pepping got stuck into just about everybody who had nursed her at the hospital. She was aged 48 in 2003 and when she signed her statement for Lieberthal she was back in the ward at the Rosebank Clinic after having repeat surgery. Her first back operation was a year earlier.

Her story was that she heard "numerous defamatory and injurious" remarks and allegations made against Lieberthal by Theunissen, Clarke and Karen Botha. She also heard all three women as well as Matron Shewan telling all Lieberthal's patients not to use him, but to rather move to Hoffmann.

"I heard these people saying Dr. Lieberthal kills and paralyses his patients. I was not prepared to entertain or listen to any defamatory, injurious remarks about Dr. Lieberthal, as in my eyes he is an angel from heaven. Dirkie (Theunissen) further told Mrs. Blackburn, who was in the ward with me, that she must go to Dr. Hoffmann because Dr. Lieberthal was useless and F…. people up, and because of my support for Dr. Lieberthal, Rosemary Clarke told me I am a *gatkruiper* (arse creeper)."

She was currently being discriminated against by the nursing staff because she had supported Lieberthal and had not moved to Hoffmann. She had developed abscesses on both buttocks because the nurses had not injected her correctly. "It has been alleged by Netcare employees that Dr. Lieberthal is paying me to say these things and to give support to him. That is clearly not the case. I would testify in any court that the aforementioned employees of Netcare have carefully planned and orchestrated Dr. Lieberthal's downfall."

Kevin Bakewell added to the number of accusations against the staff. According to him, he was told by Sisters Theunissen and Clarke and Nurse Mariba that Lieberthal's operations were never a success and some patients had come back for 13 and 14 operations. They were also supposed to have said that Lieberthal prescribed pain killers so his patients did not complain and to cover up his unsuccessful operations.

"I was told Dr. Lieberthal is never available when needed and comes approximately every five days to see his patients. Sister Dirkie Theunissen in particular said I would do better with another doctor. Dr. Lieberthal's staff was very rude and never took messages. Nurse Mariba said Dr. Lieberthal was a drug addict and was admitted to a drug rehabilitation center. At all times I was extremely happy with Dr. Lieberthal and his surgical ability." Lieberthal did a lumbar fusion operation on Bakewell who described it as a success.

I was able to find two of the people who were said to have made statements in support of Lieberthal as well as the daughter of one of them, whose story was particularly tragic.

Tertia van Eeden, a gold miner's wife, who had been a nurse herself at the Robinson private hospital in Randfontein, a heavily mined area near Johannesburg, told me that Lieberthal came to see her at her home with his lawyer, "the bloke with the long hair".

That was Advocate Goldblum, I surmised. Why had an advocate been traipsing around with his client collecting statements that were scribbled out? Lieberthal must have had a very special relationship with him because taking statements was normally the role of an advocate's instructing attorney.

The statement Van Eeden signed in 2002 made out that she was perfectly satisfied with the way Lieberthal had treated her. It was an illusion. What she told me at her home in Krugersdorp West was a horror story with much the same pattern as many of the ones that had been brought before the Health Professions Council.

A slightly built woman with a decidedly crooked spine and a limp, she had originally hurt her back by picking up patients in her work as a nurse. She had been sent to Lieberthal by Dr. Dybala, who was then based at the Robinson Hospital. She said he had sent quite a few people to Lieberthal.

Van Eeden was still in pain when I saw her and had been in theatre on 50 occasions in the last few years. She was in and out of the Rosebank Clinic from 1999 until 2004 when Lieberthal had done 35 operations on her back. A lot of these were to put in screws and remove them. On other occasions he had to clean the wound because she had got a very virulent infection at the Clinic. When I saw her, nine years after her first Lieberthal back operation, she still had a suppurating sore in her back that would not heal. Since she stopped seeing Lieberthal, a specialist in Pretoria had been treating her. Unfortunately, the skin grafts he tried would not take because of the infection.

Coming to the only part of her statement that dealt with operations

Lieberthal did on her, I said, "It says here 'On 15 August 2002 Dr. Lieberthal operated on my spine and removed a lymph node and the operation was a success'. Would that be right?"

"The first operation I had in 1999 was not a success. He did remove a lymph node in 2002 and that was successful. Every time after he operated on me I told him I still had trouble with my right leg, which was numb."

"I assume he just carried on operating?"

"Yes."

When I asked what Lieberthal had told her after each operation, she said, 'It wasn't a success'. He said that to me straight. But I thought, as he was my doctor, I must listen to him." It was amazing that even a nurse had been prepared to go on having one unsuccessful operation after another without doubting Lieberthal's competency. He really cashed in on people's belief in the infallibility of their doctor.

She said it was "definitely not true" to say that Lieberthal treated her successfully. "My back is still leaking, leaking."

I read other parts of her statement to her to see if she agreed with them. She did not know of Theunissen or Dr. Hoffmann, but she remembered Sister Priscilla saying that two patients died after Lieberthal had done 35 operations on the one person's neck and 57 operations on the other one's back. And every time she had returned to the Clinic Priscilla had told her to see another doctor.

As Van Eeden could no longer work and her husband Piet had been retrenched when the mine where he was employed closed, the couple, who had no children, appeared to be battling financially. He had a van from which he sold ice-cream.

Also in the file was a statement allegedly signed by Alison Mayers, which was one of the few that had been typed. In it she was supposed to have said that she had read the one Van Eeden had made and she confirmed much of what was in it.

But when I spoke to her at her home in Tulisa Park, a declining middle class area in the Southern part of Johannesburg where she had lived for 23 years, she said she had not signed anything. This diamond sorter for De Beers, who could no longer work, was operated on five times in a year by Lieberthal. "I had infection like you can't believe," she told me. "I nearly died."

Like Van Eeden, she still had an infected hole in her back which none of the specialists could get to heal. Her problems started with a slipped disk. "When I saw Colin Hyams, my local GP after Lieberthal had operated on me, he said, 'Oh, my God! It looks like a bomb has gone off in your back'."

A stocky woman with short cropped hair, she was bent over. Her back was evidently very sore. When I read out her statement to her, she said, "I don't know anything about that. When the crap hit the fan, let us put it that way, Dr. Lieberthal's secretary phoned me and said won't I come in and give a statement but I never said anything to anybody."

After she had given me a copy of her signature, it was clear that it was her signature on the bottom of the statement Lieberthal produced. The fishy thing about the document was that above the signature it stated, "Thus done and signed on this the 27th January 2002," when the statement itself referred to her last surgical procedure having been done by Lieberthal during August 2002. Mayers' husband Erick, an IT specialist, told me that he had no recollection of his wife having signed a statement. How did his wife's signature get on the document? Only Lieberthal would be able to clarify that.

Another so called "Affidavit" had Barbara Strydom's name on it. From what her daughter told me, she would have made a very unreliable witness had she been called to give evidence in person.

According to her statement, she had been a patient of Lieberthal's since August 2000. Aged 55, she was in the hospital to have implants removed after a successful lumbar spine fusion when she signed the document. While she was there in October 2002, Sister Clarke kept "insinuating" that Lieberthal was not competent. She was encouraged to move to another doctor.

In December 2002, Karen Botha made an appointment for her to see Hoffmann and during her consultation with this doctor he made "damning, defamatory allegations against Dr. Lieberthal". After looking at the x-rays ordered by Lieberthal, he threw them aside and said the surgical procedure Lieberthal did was "a terrible mess" and that he did not know if he could repair it. "I never went back to him as I did not like his attitude. I returned in January to see Dr. Lieberthal, as I had every confidence in him".

This confidence in her surgeon cost her dearly, from what her daughter Terry Rushmer told me. A remarkably good looking woman with the sylph-like figure of a model, Rushmer said her mother's association with Lieberthal was a "lethal concoction". He operated on her back nine times.

"Eventually it got very bad because there was a piece of metal lodged between the vertebrae which they couldn't remove," said Rushmer in her very up market home in Alberton just South of Johannesburg, where her husband Kevin had a successful compressor business. It was evidently the same kind of botched job that Cooper experienced. "She was in such agony that she went to the pain clinic in Bloemfontein. She became addicted to Pethidine and morphine. She was going from one doctor to another to get Pethidine and was injecting herself like taking sweets."

"What made her continue with Lieberthal?" I asked.

"I don't know. When she wanted to have her first op, she saw Dr. Nainkin and he refused to touch her. He said she should rather live with the pain. She was in such a self-destructive mode I really don't know what was going through her mind. If you've gone for one or let's say two operations, doesn't it register that this man doesn't know what he's doing? When he told my Mom he had to do another operation, his favorite sayings were, 'You didn't rest. It's your fault.'"

I asked her if she knew about the statement her mother was supposed to have given Lieberthal and she replied, "By that time my mother was already hooked on the drugs so I can't imagine my Mom signing that. I do know that Sister Clarke suggested she see another doctor. She was actually for it. She was saying, 'I'm being warned here', and I said, 'Mom don't go back', but she took no notice."

With difficulty Terry recalled what happened on that Friday in 2004 that will be indelibly imprinted on her mind forever. "That day my mother told me on the phone 'I hope you feel what I'm going through. You're trying to get me locked up in an asylum'. After I had picked up my kids from school, my grandmother called me. She was staying with my Mom for the weekend. She said, 'I can't cope. Your Mom is going downhill.'"

Terry got into her car and drove over to her mother's townhouse in Brackendowns not far away, unaware of the tragedy that was about to unfold. "As I got to the gate of my Mom's house I heard the shot. When I looked through into the bedroom, I could smell the gunpowder. My gran, who was about 85, hasn't got over it, although she didn't see anything. My mother shot herself here," she said, pointing under her chin.

Her husband had to break down the bedroom door to enable them to get to her mother, who died about four hours later. "Kevin was so traumatized by what he saw he had to have psychiatric treatment afterwards. Dr. Lieberthal will have his day," she added. "I believe in that."

Lieberthal also had the backing of his anesthetist, Neil Patterson, who must have been in a better position than anybody to know what Lieberthal had been up to. He had every reason to support the surgeon through whom he had evidently done very well, judging by his luxurious home complete with tennis court and pool. It was in Oaklands, a leafy suburb not far from the Rosebank Clinic, where the properties positively reeked of money.

"Since 1996, I have been the regular anaesthetist for Doctor Wynne Lieberthal on his lists being Tuesday and Thursdays," he revealed in his statement signed in February 2003. "The fact that Dr. Lieberthal was found guilty in a "trial by the media" is absolutely disgusting to say the least. Having worked with Dr. Lieberthal for so many years, I have found his approach to the care of his patients to be well-organised, precise and most professional. His surgical technique in the operating theatre has always been exceptional and his opinion and surgical expertise are widely sought by his colleagues."

Patterson had been one of Lieberthal's anesthetists from 1996 and his only one from 2001 to the date of the statement. "I have never seen him operate with a broken arm in a sling," his defense of the surgeon went on. "He did have stable, internal fixation of a fracture in early January 2002 and was fully capable, functional and made use of a specialist orthopedic assistant at this time."

His statement ended without a single reference to any nurse. It was merely a character reference that did nothing to support Lieberthal's submission to the Nursing Council that the nurses had been behaving badly.

When I went to Patterson's house to speak to him, a woman there told me he had emigrated to Australia.

Deneys Reitz, Netcare's attorneys submitted Theunissen and Clarke's responses to Lieberthal's claims. As Swart was out of the country, they undertook to get a statement from her as soon as they could. Both nurses denied the allegations that Lieberthal had made against them, and so did Karen Botha.

Clarke's response was that it was "nonsense" that the nursing staff "orchestrated the entire saga and media coverage of Sean Cooper and told him to go to Dr. Hoffmann." She never administered any injections into Pepping's buttocks and the nursing records showed that on no occasion was she treated for abscesses.

Theunissen's version was probably the closest to what actually happened. She stated, "From time to time there was concern expressed by some of the patients regarding the treatment they received from Dr. Lieberthal. The possibility of getting a second opinion was discussed by the patients among themselves. Occasionally a patient expressed to me their dissatisfaction with Dr. Lieberthal's treatment and asked about a second opinion. It was only then that I mentioned the name of Dr. Hoffmann, as he was the only neurosurgeon at the Rosebank Clinic. At all times I informed the patients that they should discuss their concerns about their treatment with Dr. Lieberthal. Samantha Mashanini's mother expressed her concern to me regarding the treatment received by her daughter from Dr. Lieberthal. I informed her that she was entitled to a second opinion, but she should go through the correct channels. It's possible I mentioned Dr. Hoffmann. I certainly never told any student nurse to tell Mrs. Mashanini that Dr. Lieberthal had "messed up" her daughter and that she should go and see Dr. Hoffmann."

Theunissen revealed Sister Nyingwa's motive for turning on her colleagues. She had also allegedly made a statement in support of Lieberthal's complaint. It appeared to be rooted in one of those black and white feuds that were not uncommon in the workplace. "While I was the unit manager, Sylvia Nyingwa was disciplined by me on a number of occasions. Afterwards she was reported as saying to staff that she will 'get me back'," Theunissen claimed.

Included in the file at the Nursing Council were statements from Cooper and Dr. Hoffmann backing the nurses. "My impression at all times was that the nursing sisters were too scared to raise any patient's complaints about Lieberthal for fear of losing their jobs," was Cooper's opinion. "No sister ever recommended that I seek assistance from Dr. Hoffmann. This was recommended to my mother via a third doctor."

Hoffmann, who had rooms at Rosebank Clinic from December 2001, read all the statements. He denied ever requesting any of the sisters to solicit patients for him or that they had in fact done this.

"I am well acquainted with Sisters Theunissen, Clarke and Swart. I have the utmost confidence in their professionalism, and in my experience, they always conducted themselves with the patient's best interests in mind. I consulted two of Dr. Lieberthal's patients, Barbara Strydom and Mark Ian Collet, in my rooms at the request of the patient or relatives of the patient. Those consultations were never, to my knowledge, arranged through any of the nursing staff.

"I deny having made any damning or defamatory remarks about Dr. Lieberthal in any consultations with Barbara Strydom or any other patient. After consulting with Collet, I informed him I was unable to assist him. I saw Sean Cooper at the request of his family in an emergency, and I also saw Jenny Musgrove, another of Dr. Lieberthal's patients in an emergency at the request of Dr. Lieberthal's locum. I deny informing Mr. Cooper that I was writing to the Board of Directors of Netcare in respect of Dr. Lieberthal and it is absurd to suggest that I have no patients except ones I have stolen from Dr. Lieberthal. I have never "stolen" patients from any doctor."

Lieberthal must have been mortified to learn that he and his supporters had made no impression at all on the Nursing Council. His complaint got treated in much the same way as many of the ones submitted to his own Medical Council by patients who felt they had been badly treated by him.

His unconvincing evidence did not help one bit. His case never even made first base. The Preliminary Investigation Committee did not consider it strong enough to warrant a Professional Conduct inquiry. It was dismissed in December 2003. Doctors evidently had no special aura as far as this nursing body was concerned.

When Netcare gave notice that it intended defending the action, Lieberthal upped the ante. He pleaded that a reasonable period of notice he should have been given was 24 months.

Each of his operations, which included consultations, generated R50 000, of which the hospital took R10 000. As he had been doing 50 operations a month, his loss of earnings over a 24-month period would have been a staggering R48-million.

Not content with that tidy sum, he added R12 799 601 for the loss of patients and profits that had been caused by what the nurses had said about him. On top of this, he put another R1-million because his "good name and reputation" had been "impaired" and he had been "humiliated" by the staff.

The court documents showed that he entered into an oral agreement in 1996 entitling him to the exclusive use of an operating theatre at the Clinic on Tuesdays and Thursdays for the entire day. His consulting rooms were given to him free of charge. The Clinic had been owned by the Clinic Holdings Group, which was taken over by Netcare in 1997.

In the interview I had with the Registrar of the Health Professions Council, Advocate Mkhize some years later, I asked him to give me some examples of what were described as "perverse incentives." These were dubious practices forbidden by the Council.

The first thing he said was, "Some come in the form of doctors being given free rooms by private hospitals."

"From my inquiries I gather it happens all the time," I said.

"Well it shouldn't."

"For instance, Lieberthal got free rooms."

"It shouldn't happen like that. They should pay rent and it must be market related. The relationship between the practitioner and the healthcare institution must be on an arm's length basis. There should be no conditions or targets for the practitioner to meet." That seemed pretty obvious to anybody who feared that they might end up in an operating assembly line, where every cut and thrust was a rush job.

"We found that in certain instances the perversity arises right there, because sometimes the private healthcare institution says, 'Oh, here are the rooms. You don't have to pay us anything. They are fully furnished. You've got all your equipment. Even the nursing sister will assist you. She's on our payroll. You don't have to do anything.' This is perverse. Then they say, 'In return for this, you must ensure a certain number of admissions to our facility.'"

Not only did Lieberthal get free rooms, but he also got all the instruments he used to do his operations paid for by the Rosebank Clinic, according to Sister Vos. "I bought all of them for him. They were very expensive and cost about R100 000."

Now if Lieberthal got his rooms and instruments for nothing he was clearly expected to perform by filling beds in the hospital, and if a theatre was allocated to him for the entire day twice a week, that was another incentive for him to keep his operating numbers up to the extremely high level that he claimed.

In 2008, I tackled Dr. Richard Friendland, who was appointed the Chief Executive Officer of Netcare in 2005, about his Group giving free rooms to doctors. He gave me the impression that he was extremely angry that I had broached such a touchy subject. "Our initial policy was not to charge rental to any of our doctors," he replied curtly. "This subsequently changed, and it is our policy to charge rental."

According to the figures Lieberthal gave to the court, he performed 600 operations a year. Even in his own sworn affidavits, he could not get his figures to correlate from one year to the next. The year before, when he tried to gag Radio 702 one of his affidavits stated that since he became an orthopedic surgeon in 1996 he had averaged "at least 350 operations per year."

Reporting on the Netcare case, The Star quoted an unnamed orthopedic surgeon, who had been practicing for 22 years and was an executive of the South African Medical Legal Society. "To the best of my knowledge he did a lot of spinal surgery and that normally takes two-and-half to three hours a case," he said. "There is no spinal surgeon in this country who will do six or seven operations every Tuesday and Thursday. And there also aren't that many patients who require that kind of surgery in the country. The profit Lieberthal claimed to have made per operation was excessive and out of line with the average orthopedic surgeon's income."

Donald Dinnie, Netcare's attorney, put Lieberthal in a catch-22 situation. He served notice on him in October 2004 to produce 93 documents relevant to the case. They involved the entire volume of his dubious past, including all Lieberthal's unprofessional charges. He was also asked to bring the books of account for his practice from 1 January 1995 to the date of the notice as well as his income tax returns for the same period.

In May 2004, the Receiver of Revenue obtained a judgment against Lieberthal in the Johannesburg Magistrate's Court for non-payment of tax amounting to R114 420. It was anybody's guess as to what his books of account and income tax returns might have revealed.

He claimed the documents were privileged. No wonder he didn't want them disclosed. That could have invited another media feeding frenzy. Considerable argument followed about their discovery and in December 2004 Dinnie stated in an affidavit: "I respectfully draw the attention to this Honourable Court that this matter has been set down for hearing on 1 March 2005 and the Defendant is being severely prejudiced in its preparation for trial by the Plaintiff's failure to make proper discovery." He accused Lieberthal's legal team of not complying with the Rules of Court.

It looked as though Dinnie had brought off a brilliant coup because a settlement was reached just before the case was due to come before court.

According to The Star, Michael Sacks, the chairperson of Netcare, refused to give details of the settlement. However, Cottrell told me he doubted if Lieberthal got paid anything. "While I was at Rosebank, a patient arrived from Zimbabwe with R70 000. He gave it all to Lieberthal, but part of it was supposed to be for the hospital and Lieberthal refused to part with the clinic's share. I think Netcare was countersuing him for the money when he was claiming against them."

In a June 2004 article headed "Dr. Jekyll or Mr. High", Noseweek magazine said of Lieberthal, "A pill-popping orthopaedic surgeon, with Walter Mitty fantasies and a penchant for dubious insurance claims, would be enough to send a chill up anyone's spine." Elsewhere it reported, "Usually reliable sources suggest Lieberthal has run out of money and consequently out of lawyers." His cases against The Star and Primedia just petered out.

Whether anybody at the Medical Council saw this article that exposed Lieberthal and the other doctors involved in the insurance frauds I don't know. It certainly never took any action against them for this.

Lieberthal's efforts to extract money through the courts were very costly gambles that never paid off, at a time when he could have done with the money, as he claimed he and his family was virtually destitute. He was already pleading poverty a year earlier. In the middle of 2003, The Star got a judgment against him for costs totaling R38 152. Deon van Dijk, the Deputy Sheriff, served a copy of the writ of execution on Lieberthal personally at his Johannesburg home. It was a demand for payment of the amount involved, plus his costs of R438.

"Wynne Lieberthal informed me," he said, "that he has no money, property or assets whereby to satisfy this warrant or any portion thereof. He declared that all the assets on the property belong to his wife and they are married with an anti-nuptial contract."

Their assets were not jointly owned but belonged to whoever's name they were in. So his wife's goods could not be seized to satisfy a judgment against the doctor, a very convenient arrangement in the circumstances.

To compound his court room disappointments, the Health Professions Council was at long last doing what it should have done ages ago; taking action to protect patients from getting maimed by this scalpel-happy surgeon, who appeared to be in the business purely for money.

Would Lieberthal once again be able to convince the sympathetic Council that it was misguided and that he had done nothing wrong?

Chapter 17

After His Blood

When the Health Professions Council's disciplinary hearing finally got under way in earnest in January 2004, after several adjournments, Lieberthal's defense team began the proceedings in a mind-boggling fashion that could only have surprised the members of the three-man Committee that was there to try him. They were Dr. Piet Barnard, the Chairman, who was sitting with Professor Shunmugam Govender, head of the orthopedic department at the KwaZulu-Natal University's Medical School, and Dr. "Obie" Oberholster, a retired general practitioner.

Barnard, at aged 68, still had his own GP practice in Pretoria. Like Oberholster, he spent quite a lot of his time on committees of the Council's disciplinary inquiries. Sitting with them, to advise them on points of law, was 74-year-old "SAS" Strauss, a retired law professor whose specialty had been criminal and medical law. He had written numerous reference books on medical and nursing law. The Council's expert witness was Professor Mkhuleli "Mac" Lukhele. His expertise was spinal surgery. He was in charge of the Spine Unit at Garankuwa Hospital from 1990 until 2002, when he was appointed Chief Specialist at the Orthopedic Department of the Johannesburg Hospital. There he established a Spinal Disorder Unit.

The way the hearing started established the "bend over backwards to be fair to Dr. Lieberthal" character of the entire proceedings. The interests of the long suffering, permanently impaired patients, who had been lined up to give evidence, were relegated almost to Ward Z.

Lieberthal appeared in the auditorium at the premises of the Health Professions Council in Pretoria. He was fighting to prevent his career umbilical cord from being severed by allegations contained in eight charges of unprofessional conduct. These were:

1. That during February 1998 he fused part of Martha Lawson's spine at a certain level when the operation was not necessary and that when he did this, he failed to do a fusion which should have been done at another level. On a third occasion, he did another unnecessary fusion on her in March 1998.

2. That during May 1999 when he operated on Florence Souter's spine, he

failed to remove disc material and other tissue. In the first of two operations he did on her in June 1999, he failed to identify or properly repair a cerebral-spinal fluid leak with the result that the second operation would not have been necessary had he done the job properly in the first place.

3. That during June 1999 he performed a laminectomy and a fusion on Jan Visagie and in so doing inserted unnecessary hardware without properly securing the pedicle screws and that during November 1999 he did corrective surgery on him which would not have been necessary had he done the first one properly.

4. That during the period January 1999 and February 2000 he did five back operations on Maria Whitaker and that he failed to secure the screws properly in the second one. That the third, fourth, and fifth operations would have been unnecessary had he done the second one correctly. And that he left the patient with an incorrect curvature of the spine. The last part of this charge was that he improperly arranged for the patient's husband to give her Pethidine injections when the man was not trained or authorized to do this.

5. That he did two operations on Teresa Broda between September 1997 and February 2001, when the first one was not necessary. That he told her before the first operation that she required immediate surgery because she had cancer or tuberculosis on her spine when he had no grounds for saying this. He was also accused of failing to properly investigate her condition and treat her conservatively before deciding to operate. An additional allegation was that having decided to operate on the first occasion, he inserted a standalone cage when he knew or ought to have known that this would not achieve the required fusion.

6. That during June and July 2001 he operated twice on Edward Mileham. In the first operation, he was charged with putting in pedicle screws of the wrong diameter, with the result that they had to be replaced in the second operation.

7. That between October 1997 and October 2001 he operated four times on Elizabeth Elliot's back when he should have known that the more he operated on her, the less the chance was of a successful result. He was also accused of putting pedicle screws in the wrong place from the first operations onwards and then having to do further operations to try and correct the situation.

8. That he did six spine operations on Irene Dos Santos between January and June 2002. During the first operation, it was claimed he missed a degenerated disc and then did a second operation, which would not have been necessary had the first one been done correctly. During the second operation, he was accused of allowing the wound to become septic with the result that she had to have multiple operations to clean it out. Also, he was allegedly responsible for her becoming bed ridden. The last allegation was that he refused to communicate with the family of this elderly woman regarding her treatment, condition, and progress.

Only four of the people mentioned in the charges were on the list of 32 submitted by the three surgeons nearly four years earlier. They were Lawson, Souter, Whitaker, and Elliot, all of whom had been seen by Dr. Craig.

The arrogant surgeon pleaded not guilty to all the charges. After all, a spinal specialist of his caliber could not possibly have botched this many operations and behaved in such a callous way.

With Lieberthal's unbelievable luck that had protected him so far from any serious consequences over a period of nearly two decades, he only had to answer a mere seven charges. The eighth one was abandoned and the Medical Council that had treated him so leniently for so many years once again turned a blind eye to all the other complaints that had been piling up against him. It was apparently working on the assumption that, as the worst penalty it could impose was to strike a doctor off the register, it had brought enough charges against Lieberthal to accomplish that.

A year earlier, the HPCSA revealed that the 32 complaints against Lieberthal from the orthopedic trio of doctors had been discovered. Two months before that, in October 2002, it put the number of complaints being investigated at 28. If Press reports were to be believed, there had been an incredible 60, possibly as many as 70 complaints, which was a South African record for the number made to the Medical Council against the same doctor.

How did the Council manage to whittle down this vast number to so few that warranted being incorporated in a charge sheet? Did anybody actually go through the entire list or were the eight just chosen more or less at random? If this short list was considered sufficient, was the Council being fair to all the other people, who might have had very good cases and were waiting for the Council's decision before deciding whether or not to sue Lieberthal for damages in a civil court?

Complaints to the HPCSA don't cost the complainant anything. So it could be a great help to have a positive finding of negligence from the Council before going to lawyers, especially if you don't have much money and want them to work on a contingency basis. It gives them the right incentive because they won't take your case on a no-win, no-pay basis if they are not very confident of succeeding.

The only plus on the Council's side was that it had hired a big gun to represent it against the doctor, who was high profile for all the wrong reasons. Senior Counsel Danny Berger was assisted by Advocate Ngwako Maenetje. Berger's considerable experience included appearing at the Truth and Reconciliation Commission, where apartheid sinners had been expected to confess their dastardly deeds.

The Council had evidently decided that for this case, which they instituted very belatedly, they needed to be represented by senior counsel and a junior rather than have it handled by somebody from its own legal department. Perhaps the viper-like vitriolic behavior of the doctor, who was clearly not going to admit to anything, no matter how overwhelming the evidence, had made the Council wary of him. Perhaps it was felt that he would engage the best legal team available and the Council would have to match, if not better, it. Or perhaps it was the glare of publicity that had provoked the Council into this show of force.

As it was, Lieberthal's legal team had no fearful standing about it. He did things on the cheap. He began with Advocate David Goldblum, his longtime legal adviser. He was by no means as high powered as a senior counsel and as the hearing proceeded it became increasingly puzzling as to why Lieberthal had engaged an advocated with his tenuous background to try and save his skin, in a case in which his entire career hung in the balance.

Dos Santos died before the hearing got underway. This, according to Berger, was not the reason why this charge had been withdrawn, but because "there was a lack of sufficient evidence, in our view, to prosecute that charge."

Advocate Goldblum kicked off the hearing by saying, "In terms of the regulations it might not particularly state that the defense can read a statement at this point. However, due to the nature of this entire matter and all the media hype and publicity and everything else, all extremely damaging against my client, the defense, with leave of the Committee, wishes to read this statement into the record. This is a statement made by my client."

To say that his request was unconventional would be putting it mildly. Whoever heard of a case of this nature that began with the defense?

Without waiting for the Committee's consent, he just carried on reading Lieberthal's grievances. This was the first of many instances that were to show how weak the Committee was when it came to controlling Lieberthal's tactics that were transparently aimed at putting off judgment day forever, if possible.

"For the past sixteen months I have tried to no avail to have my voice heard in this Council, my own professional body," Goldblum began. "It ludicrously claims to guide the profession, yet it was the culprit in chief for these sixteen months. Advocate Mkhize, the CEO, has refused to take my phone calls or return messages and has refused to reply to written correspondence submitted on my behalf by Advocate Goldblum, myself, and attorney, Krawitz, all of which are on record. In sixteen months, he has spoken to me once, when I got through to him on his direct line."

The Chairman looked as though he was dying to put a stop to this attack on the Council's registrar and chief executive officer, but nobody did anything, so Goldblum read on.

Complaints about Mkhize's "blatant unprofessional behaviour" were reported to various Council members. Lieberthal also spoke to Professor Lukhele, who expressed his disenchantment with the manner in which matters were being handled and had considered resigning as the orthopedic consultant to the Health Professions Council.

The tactless surgeon then alternated his attack between the Council in general, which of course included the three people who were trying him and

Mkhize, who he put in the same category as the wild dogs of the media, which had been trailing him for months on end.

"You see, Mr. Chairman, my case has been more than a game and a power play to members of the Council. For the past sixteen months, I have been unable to work mainly due to my trial by the media and continued obstruction and harassment by the HPC. This was despite not being found guilty on a single charge as yet."

The surgeon was doing his usual trick; laying the blame for his predicament on anybody but himself. "Attempts at finding work have been totally unsuccessful, mainly due to Council's obstruction. One such example was a post offered to me at East London at a state hospital. A certificate of good standing was requested after I fully informed them of my current circumstances and pending cases."

He had been refused the certificate even with an endorsement and he was "highly suspicious" at the ease with which the media was able to access Mkhize. Each time Mkhize made a media statement it had been "fundamentally wrong." He believed that an "improper relationship existed between the HPC and the media."

Lieberthal lamented the fact that his story had run as radio and newspaper headlines for almost two weeks, with numerous subsequent articles. "I wish to point out that this coverage exceeded that given to September 11, the Bali bombings and was on a par with the US/Iraq conflict."

Magotle, the Council's media liaison officer, had constantly denied that there had been anything wrong with the way the Council had dealt with the media. But the day before the last hearing there was once again "damaging and inaccurate media coverage in The Star and on Radio 702." When Lieberthal spoke to Magotle, who he thought was a reasonable person, Magotle denied knowledge of a media release by the HPC. "Imagine my utter dismay when I heard him on Radio 702 and in the later edition of The Star on the same day he was quoted."

Describing the damaging effects all the publicity had on his family, Lieberthal's version went on. "I have five children. One was writing matric in 2003 and one is disabled. Imagine, if you can, for one minute, their pain. My wife has likewise had to suffer the same humiliation. Things have become so unbearable that my daughter, who is in a position academically to choose anything she wishes, has rather left the country. Of course, I am now not in a position to afford university fees in any event. My children's schooling is unpaid. My house bond has been unpaid for a year. I have had to surrender all my policies and sell all items of value."

Continuing to try and get support for his cause, the thick-skinned surgeon could not help lacing his words with more insults that belittled the organisation represented by the Committee in front of him. "All my staff, five families, sir, four from disadvantaged backgrounds, have been dismissed because I can't pay them. I have been stripped of all my personal dignity and my reputation has been utterly and totally destroyed by the media, which has been ably assisted by the Council, prior to any guilty finding, whatsoever. Within the medical fraternity, my integrity is now questioned and patients will have nothing to do with me. The irony, sir, is that if I am found not guilty of all charges, my practice and career of twenty-three years will have been destroyed. I have been deprived of all income for 16 months by the circus that calls itself the media, and, should I be found guilty, I would have already started my sentence sixteen months ago, before I even had the benefit of a trial."

He complained that no one had apologized nor explained the "see-sawing number of cases" he was allegedly guilty of. "The number, according to Mr. Mkhize, has varied from over seventy to eighty."

The Star and Radio 702 were the only two sections of the media that carried his story with "intensity and venom, not yet seen in medical practice in South Africa." His own professional body, the HPCSA, had given him "absolutely no support" and had refused to reply to written correspondence, let alone telephone messages; the major culprits being Mr. Mkhize and Mr. Coetzer. Johan Coetzer was the senior manager in charge of Professional Boards. He left in April 2006.

Lieberthal had telephonic conversations with Professor Becker and Professor Mariba without them being able or willing to assist him. I assumed that the Becker he was talking about was Len Becker, the President of the old South African Medical and Dental Council, who had been exceptionally lenient with Lieberthal twelve years earlier when he was under supervision because of his drug abuse. Professor Thanyani Mariba, I knew, was an important member of the HPCSA.

"I have been subjected to humiliating psychiatric evaluations and urine drug testing without explanation, despite all tests being negative. Two days prior to me receiving written notice of such testing, Regan Thaw phoned my attorney, Mr. Krawitz, requesting information pertaining to this. How on earth could he have known about this?"

Goldblum paused as if he was uncertain as to whether he should read out the last part, which presumably he had no part in drafting. Then he went on parroting his master's words. "Finally, I would like to say that all of you representing this body should be deeply ashamed of yourselves by your actions and lack of actions. And I trust that the Human Rights Commission will deal with this body and its members in an appropriate manner in due course."

Lieberthal followed this with what was probably the most ludicrous statement he had made in view of what he had written up to that stage.

"I wish to state I have no dispute whatever with any of the tribunal members. I know Professor Govender and I have nothing but the highest regards for him as a colleague and, more importantly, as a decent human being."

A credit controller who worked for Philips South Africa was the first to give evidence led by Advocate Berger. Elizabeth Elliott was forty-four in October 1997 when Lieberthal did the first of four operations on her back.

After the last operation, which was done in June 2002, she concluded Lieberthal was not the expert he was made out to be. That was when she wrote a letter of complaint to the HPCSA.

She explained that she first went to see him because of pains in her legs and lower back. He recommended a fusion straight away.

After being in hospital for a few days, she was discharged, even though she was still in a great deal of pain. Lieberthal prescribed "a lot of medication" for the pain and to enable her to sleep. The x-rays showed six screws and a plate had been inserted in her back.

"About a year later, in August 1998, the pain had become very intense," she wrote, "because two screws in my back had actually broken." A second operation followed to replace these, but all six were actually replaced. "The bottoms of the two broken screws were left in my back as they were too firmly lodged to be removed."

The pain continued. So, in August 1999, she had a third operation as the fusion had been unsuccessful and had to be redone. During each operation, bone was taken from her right hip, which further added to her pain. The affected muscles went into spasm regularly.

Lieberthal did the last operation because one of the screws had gone through the bone. This had been aggravating the nerves. He felt the fusion would hold, so he decided to remove the screws. "But when I woke up after the operation I discovered the screws had been replaced once again, even though the fusion was now fully grown."

Giving evidence at the inquiry, she said that two or three years before her first operation she had a fall. She was treated and nothing significant was found. Her back ache continued and she was given medication at a clinic.

Her mother-in-law had been successfully treated by Lieberthal, and that was why she went to see him.

She had been unaware that Lieberthal was going to put screws in her back until she saw them on the x-rays. "Had my family known about this, I'm sure they would have stopped me having the op in the first place," she said.

Every time she woke up after an operation, there was a bag full of screws next to her bed. The first time there were four, plus two tops. The second time there were six and there were also six the third time. After the fourth operation Lieberthal told her that at a later stage he would have to fuse the vertebra "higher up."

She told Berger that she refused to have another operation because people were being retrenched at her firm and they were trying to force her to go on to "temporary disability", which she could not afford. "Unfortunately, I have to work," she added. "I'm too scared to have any more surgery."

In reply to further questions from Berger, she said Lieberthal "definitely" did not give her any conservative treatment before her first operation. He admitted her "very quickly."

She was still in a lot of pain. "It has never gone away. I don't know if it will ever go. At the moment, I practically live on pain tablets. Sometimes it becomes so bad I have to go to my GP and let him give me an injection, Voltaren or some concoction he makes up."

At the resumption of the inquiry the following day, Goldblum again raised the subject of the media, which Lieberthal's team had made such a feature of during the hearing. Lieberthal was taking every opportunity to prolong things, with the more red herrings the better.

Goldblum's criticism this time was that, in a 702 broadcast about the hearing Thaw had said, among other things, "The Council believes Lieberthal is guilty." He asked for some kind of assurance that this kind of thing would be stopped. "It's just like trying to stem an avalanche. It's absolutely impossible." He blamed the Council's officials for continually "slating" Lieberthal through the media and he believed his client could not get a fair trial if this kind of publicity was allowed to continue.

Responding Berger accepted the broadcast was wrong but maintained the Committee could not control what happened outside the proceedings. If Lieberthal had a complaint again 702, the correct place to deal with it was the High Court. "There can be no doubt whatsoever that Dr. Lieberthal is getting a fair trial," he added

It was like a tennis match with the Committee hearing the same tired arguments going backwards and forwards, seemingly forever. Lieberthal must have been laughing at how easily he and his counsel were able to divert the proceedings from the real issues.

Goldblum had to be told to move on after he had once again repeated the same question in a different form. He had not got very far when he said, "Sorry, at this point I need to have an adjournment. I need to have some medication."

Lieberthal explained that Goldblum was "indisposed" and would not be in a position to continue that afternoon. The Committee had no option other than to put the inquiry off until the following day. Another delay was just what Lieberthal must have wanted. Was this why he had engaged a very sick advocate?

Teresa Broda, a Polish woman, was another of Lieberthal's patients who was so dissatisfied with the treatment she received that she sent a letter to the HPCSA in October 2002. Her distressing Lieberthal experience began in 1997.

She gave evidence at the hearing through a Polish interpreter. In reply to questions by Berger, she said that, when she consulted Lieberthal for the first time, he saw something wrong on the MRI scan, but he was not sure if it was cancer or a tumor. "But my situation is very serious, so he said I would have to be operated on immediately. I started crying because I had only started working seven months before this and I was afraid that I would be dismissed if I had long sick leave. He said my health situation was so serious that within three months I would stop walking. 'If you were my wife, I would operate on you today,' he told me when I asked if the operation could be delayed." Three days later, he operated on her spine.

Trying to find out how thorough Lieberthal had been before deciding to do this, Berger established that she was not sent to any other doctors and nor did she have any further tests to show if the growth was cancerous.

On the second day after the operation, she was "breathing like a fish" because there was a hole in her back from where a rib had been removed for her fusion. She was very relieved when Lieberthal told her the growth was not malignant, as that had been her biggest fear.

His assistant for this operation was Jon Patricios, a 28-year-old GP who worked at the Sport Medicine Centre in the same building as Lieberthal's consulting rooms. They were friends at one stage, however it did not stop the surgeon doing the dirty on him and, as was so often the case with our greedy specialist, money was the cause of the fallout. Lieberthal didn't pay him.

When I spoke to him about it, he chortled before saying, "It's an episode in my past. At the time it was an issue, but now I don't need to get involved in that sort of stuff."

Another doctor also struggled to get his money for assisting the high-earning surgeon with his operations: his long-time friend and fellow con artist, Attila Szabo. He had to go to the Council for Conciliation, Mediation and Arbitration, a statutory body that resolves labor disputes. The skinflint was forced to pay Szabo, who was an orthopedic surgeon living in Cape Town when I spoke to him.

Broda went back to Lieberthal in January 2001 because she was still having so much pain. After he told her that the "bones did not grow together", she wanted to get a second opinion. The persuasive surgeon talked her out of it by saying that any doctor could see that there was a fracture of the vertebra. He promised she would "definitely" have no pain after her second operation. Like many of his predictions, this proved to be very wide of the mark.

"When I woke up after the second operation, I felt a pronounced pain in my left leg and left side of my lower back," she told Berger. "I have never experienced such pain. I started screaming that something was wrong. I will not be able to walk any more, I kept telling them. Then they gave me a tranquilizing injection. When Lieberthal arrived, he said the pain was due to a bladder infection, and he gave me tablets for this." She stopped seeing him three months later because she no longer trusted him. She was able to work, but still had to take painkillers.

Eddie Mileham was coming to the end of his professional boxing career in 1978. He had been the holder of the South African white lightweight title. In those days of apartheid, there were black and white champions.

The African Ring magazine said of him, "Eddie's magnificent conditioning and dedication made him a fearless champion in an era of exceptional lightweights."

In June of that year, he had gone across the border to Salisbury (now Harare) in Rhodesia (now Zimbabwe) to fight Tadios Fisher. At that stage, Fisher had taken several unsuccessful cracks at the Rhodesian lightweight and welterweight titles, although he did finally succeed in taking the welterweight crown a year later. Unlike South Africa, Rhodesia did not have segregated championships.

Fisher was also nearing the end of a career that had spanned ten years, double the time that Mileham had been a professional pugilist. This was a run-of-the-mill fight with no title involved.

"Rhodesia still had a white government then," Mileham told me nearly thirty years after the fight, "because you could walk around freely and Salisbury was a beautiful town."

Surprisingly, in the lounge of his flat in the southern suburbs of Johannesburg, there was little evidence of his boxing achievements. On one wall, there was just a framed photograph of Mileham, together with a copy of a title fight program. It was when he lost a non-title fight to Jan Snyders on the same bill in 1973, when South Africa's Arnold Taylor knocked out Romeo Anaya of Mexico to win the World Boxing Association Bantamweight title. There were no signs of any trophies or other memorabilia.

Now aged fifty-two, Mileham still looked extremely fit, much like the photograph on the wall. His hair style had not changed since the seventies. It was still shoulder length and his sideburns were still as long as they were in those days, only now streaks of grey were creeping in everywhere.

The Salisbury fight was held at the National Sports Centre and, after eight bruising rounds, the referee raised Mileham's hand to signify that he had won on points. That did it. All hell broke loose.

"Fisher was quite a strong guy," Mileham told me, "and I said to my trainer Joe Williams, 'I'll fight Tadios Fisher, he's nothing'. I had prepared well. I underestimated him. It was touch and go for both of us. I think I had the better of him, though. I was a bit too classy for him. When they announced that I was the winner, the crowd of about five hundred blacks went mad. Shoo! They stormed the ring. There were just us three whites, me, my trainer, and my assistant trainer inside a ring which was moving up and down. They were trying to tip the whole thing over with us in it." He was grabbed by his trainer, who rushed him straight to the airport, and Mileham changed out of his boxing togs on the plane.

To calm the enraged mob somebody had the presence of mind to announce, "Please, ladies and gentlemen, there has been a terrible mistake. The winner is Tadios Fisher."

"And that's how it stands in the record books today," Mileham said. "That was by far my worst experience."

In 1979, Mileham got a job with the Johannesburg City Municipality as a plumber. It was some time after he had stopped fighting professionally that the fight of his life really began. He revealed what happened when he gave evidence at Lieberthal's disciplinary hearing.

He was still working when he had an operation done by Dr. Snykers for lower back pain. Afterwards, it got worse and his wife, Mary, suggested he should go to Lieberthal this time. "She had an operation by him and she said he's very good," he told Berger.

Lieberthal operated on him for the first time in June 2001 and again not long afterwards. After the first one, Mileham had a "burning sensation" in his back. One leg was "numb and cold." Lieberthal put this down to a blood clot. Then, when he looked at Mileham's x-rays and MRI scan, Lieberthal realized that two of the screws he had put in were too long. They had to be removed because they were pressing on a nerve.

"Did Dr. Lieberthal tell you what he was going to do in this second operation?" Berger asked.

"Not at all. I still thought it was a blood clot. When I woke up, Dr. Lieberthal was standing next to me with the screws. He said, 'Here are the screws I had to remove.'"

Why did Lieberthal have this macabre practice of presenting his patients with the screws he had removed from their backs, like some kind of trophy, as if he was proud of his expertise? It was rather like when you take your car to the garage for a service and they leave you with the old parts that they have replaced as proof of what they have done. Perhaps some doctors are just mechanics by another name?

This scared his patients, especially those who were told they needed another operation. It didn't seem to concern this popular specialist that by doing this, he was giving them metallic proof of his shoddy workmanship.

"Let's come to how you are feeling now," said Berger.

"I have still got much back pain every day. I cannot sit or stand too long and my left foot, at the bottom, is still numb; it is dead."

Professor Lukhele's assessment made Lieberthal's denials of negligence look more and more unlikely. He believed that surgery for Mileham had not been indicated at all. He would have treated him conservatively for at least three months before deciding to operate.

Mileham's fight of his life will continue for the rest of his days. Dr. Wynne Lieberthal, spinal surgeon extraordinaire, had seen to that.

Mrs. Souter had been referred to Lieberthal by Dr. Dybala, who saw her at the Robinson Hospital. Her left leg was "on fire" and she could not stand. She was taken to the Rosebank Clinic by ambulance where Lieberthal operated on her back on three occasions over a two-month period in 1999.

About three weeks after the first operation her foot "ballooned and became extremely sensitive" so she was readmitted to the Clinic. "I was crying in the ward because I could sense something had gone horribly wrong. Dr. Lieberthal sent me for another MRI scan. Afterwards, when he came back to my bed and told me I needed another operation, I thought, "Oh no, I cannot believe this." He said he had not removed an entire disc and I had probably dislodged the remaining bit in a fit of coughing. He now had to remove it as it was pressing against a nerve."

She denied ever having had a cough.

After the second operation, fluid kept seeping out of the wound. Those present did their best to hide a snigger as she said, "Yes, and my bed was facing the entrance. Then I realized everybody could see me and I didn't have my panties on. The fluid was all over the bed. I was just left in that state."

She saw Dr. Lieberthal again in September 1999 because she was still having "terrible pain." Looking at her new set of x-rays he said, "Your fusion is growing beautifully but you won't be able to contact me in the near future because I'm going away." She never went back to him after that.

Subsequently, she saw various doctors. Dr. Fourie, a neurosurgeon at the Robinson Hospital, took away the "electric shocks" she was still getting in her back.

When he first examined her, he said, "Mrs. Souter you have been panel beaten." He added, "In my opinion, you did not need a fusion." In August 2000, the fusion was redone in the Wilgeheuwel Hospital at Roodepoort by orthopedic surgeon, Dr. Oosthuizen, and Dr. Wasserman, a neurosurgeon, because it had come loose. Having another go at Lieberthal, she said, "Their diagnosis was that the original fusion had not taken because of an infection I had when Dr. Lieberthal discharged me. Today my back is much better. I do have pain but it is bearable as I take as much as six pain killers a day. I no longer have pain in my leg and I am regaining movement in my ankle. My foot is still paralyzed."

Her anger boiled to the surface when Berger asked, "How do you feel towards Dr. Lieberthal now?"

"I absolutely hate that man. I just want to kill him."

The Chairman asked Goldblum to begin his cross-examination of Souter. Looking sickly and in pain he replied, "No sir, I am not in a position at all to continue. I am totally incapacitated, which I explained to my colleague earlier."

A brief delay followed. At the resumption, Advocate Harold Knopp appeared, saying he was now acting for Lieberthal.

Knopp then disclosed the secret about Goldblum that had been kept from the Committee. He could not continue because of a 20-year long illness, which caused him severe pain with bowel and bladder problems. He had been advised by his specialist to withdraw from the proceedings to avoid further damage to his health.

At that stage, the Committee trying Lieberthal had been on the go intermittently for seven months. An unavoidable delay was caused when Professor Lukhele was shot and wounded in an attempted car hijacking.

Knopp's first move when he took over the defense in January 2004 was to plead poverty on behalf of his client and ask for another adjournment. "Advocate Goldblum had been acting on a pro amico basis and it would be difficult, if not impossible, to get a replacement on this basis," he said. "The further difficulty is that Dr. Lieberthal has no funds to engage legal representation."

He then made the farcical suggestion that the Medical Council should pay for Lieberthal's defense. "Alternatively, the Legal Aid Board or some private institutions may possibly fund his legal defense. It is my respectful submission that, because this matter is serious and complex, Dr. Lieberthal would be severely prejudiced and would not receive a fair hearing, if he were to be deprived of legal representation."

"Everyone involved in the hearing," Berger replied, "had attempted to make the necessary allowances so that Advocate Goldblum could be part of the proceedings. But there was also no doubt that Dr. Lieberthal had known that this advocate was not in a position to run this litigation. And what steps were taken by Dr. Lieberthal to seek other legal representation? We know of none."

He contended that Lieberthal would not suffer any prejudice by not being assisted by Goldblum because "it has been plain for all to see that almost every question, almost every objection, that has come from Advocate Goldblum originated in the mouth of Dr. Lieberthal." Goldblum had been reading out a whole series of questions written by Lieberthal and there were times when he could not read the doctor's writing.

At last Berger focused on the almost forgotten aspect of the inquiry. "All this time we have been talking about the interests of Dr. Lieberthal, but there are also the interests of the Council in obtaining finality in this matter." He referred to the note doctors charged with misconduct received. This stipulated that they could be legally represented, but if they did not make arrangements for this timeously or did not appear, the hearing could still go ahead.

The Committee eventually decided not to grant any of Dr. Lieberthal's requests and adjourned to the following day. As they were putting their documents away, Knopp surprised everyone by saying, "I will not be here tomorrow. My mandate was merely to bring the application for postponement and legal funding."

Lieberthal's next move made nonsense of his destitute story, unless he had suddenly found a rich benefactor. He launched an urgent High Court action in Pretoria to have the Committee's decision overturned. They were not going to get the better of Dr. Wynne Lieberthal, the well-known orthopedic surgeon, who specialized in spinal disorders.

In the pathetic affidavit, he submitted to the Court he argued that he would be unable to conduct his own defense adequately. "I have been advised that I must proceed with the hearing on my own, with or without legal representation. My entire career and livelihood is at stake," was his final play for compassion. He maintained the Medical Council had been unreasonable in denying him a postponement, as this would in no way have prejudiced the Council.

A compromise was reached at the Court a day later and accepted by Lieberthal. The effect of this was that the hearing would resume with Lieberthal cross-examining Souter before the matter would be adjourned to allow the doctor to brief new council.

Lieberthal, the legal ignoramus, was now on his own, up against a formidable prosecuting team. He must have felt like some of his patients did when they struggled to decipher the complexities of the medical jargon involved in back operations.

The hearing continued with the doctor, who had maimed so many people, being wet-nursed once again. The ever helpful Strauss advised the Committee that, as Lieberthal was not legally represented, they should "not hesitate" to assist him in asking questions. The Professor also asked to be allowed to intervene, where necessary, to help Lieberthal with legal aspects of his case. He conceded that it was "unusual for a legal assessor like myself to be assisting the defense."

Lieberthal was finally told he could cross-examine Souter with more reassuring words from the Chairman, who said, "Dr. Lieberthal, do not hesitate to ask assistance of Professor Strauss at any point."

Then the fun really started. Anybody who might have been about to doze off would have found themselves alerted by a new, very different, verbal battle. It was such a contrast to the ultra-polite banter of the advocates arguing the case up to that stage.

Souter might have been the submissive patient prepared to take Lieberthal's word for everything when he was treating her, but on this new stage, she was a different woman altogether. A sharp-witted spitfire, she had clearly come there to give Lieberthal some of her own medicine.

Without the lifebelt of his legal adviser, Lieberthal struggled to keep afloat in this unfamiliar setting. Unlike in a hospital, he was no longer being treated with the reverence of a God who could do no wrong.

He came off a very bad second best in his efforts to show Souter up as an unreliable witness. At times, she threatened to walk out after several clashes with her former surgeon.

At his smarmy best, Lieberthal began, "When you gave evidence two days ago, you were very angry. You stated you hated me and wanted to kill me, but, unfortunately, you are going to have to answer some questions before you can put that plan into action."

Not easily intimidated, she replied, "Well, if I had planned to do it, I would have done it long ago."

When he asked her to tell him the "sequence of events that you think occurred." she came back at him with this smart Alec reply, "Which I think occurred, or really occurred?"

On another occasion, he got her going by saying that Dr. Dybala and other people who had seen her, had confirmed that she was an "extremely tense and highly strung woman." She screamed back, "You are defaming me, saying I'm impatient and highly strung."

"You have already demonstrated this," Lieberthal retorted. "You wanted to walk out within one minute."

"Because you nearly killed me," she shot back.

He questioned her about her claim that she woke up after the operation feeling like a "bionic woman," although she said he had not told her he was going to put screws in her back. "I have screws in my own back and ten in my left humerus and you can't feel one of them," he said.

Interestingly, two years later he had a failed bone graft removed from his arm at the Sunninghill, which was another hospital in the Netcare Group. He didn't pay the hospital's bill of R9 143, resulting in a 2004 Magistrate's Court judgment against him for a R4 124 debt, so it was difficult to understand why he was given credit once again, especially as he was kicked out of the Rosebank Clinic, which was in the same group. In 2009, Netcare's legal department was still looking for him because the summons they issued in connection with the R9 143 was returned. The hospital then blacklisted him with the largest credit bureau in the country.

Souter came up with some more repartee when Lieberthal asked her to explain the significance of her statement that she had been awake when she was transferred from the operating table to the trolley after her third operation.

"The relevance is; it is very bad care of the patients. I was uncomfortable and in a lot of pain. Surely I must not wake up as I'm tossed from the theatre table onto the trolley."

"Well, with all due respects, you do not get tossed from the one to the other. Secondly, whose responsibility do you think the anesthetic is? There was an anesthetist who chose to wake you up when he did. It had, quite frankly, nothing to do with me when he woke you."

She was enjoying herself. "So I was not under your care? I was not your patient?"

"I am telling you that he may have chosen, for whatever reason, to wake you while you were on the table. The anesthetist was a specialist and it was his judgment, his call."

Lieberthal seemed oblivious to the fact that his quick-witted adversary had bettered him in most of these skirmishes, and even if he won the odd round, he had no chance of disproving his guilt by continuing to cross-examine her.

He was only making his position worse.

Emphasizing that he would not have told her to take as much Lentogesic as she wanted to, he said he was well aware of prescribing precautions. This set her off again.

"Oh really? I am still addicted to that stuff, thanks to you."

"Yes, I'm sure it's all my doing, Mrs. Souter. You said a lot of things which are extremely damaging to me and I am having difficulty now in getting to the core of the truth of this complaint."

"You have difficulty, but the people you operated on must not complain?"

"We are not talking about people. We are talking about you, Mrs. Souter. You and your evidence."

"So if I have got a problem, I have got an attitude, hey?"

Strauss blew his whistle again. "Let's just take it easy, Mrs. Souter. The Committee is hearing your evidence so will you please respond to the questions. We would like to avoid recriminations."

"He started it so I had to react," she retorted, addressing the Committee. "He accused me of damaging his reputation."

Defending himself, Lieberthal said, "No, I did not say that. I said you have said damaging things like 'panel beating' which just happened to hit the media headlines, together with 'hating him' and wanting to 'kill him'. They were in the paper and on 702 news. You had your photograph taken for the newspaper."

"That is not damaging to you having my photo in the newspaper," she hit back, outflanking the surgeon.

"My point is that you knew about the newspaper and the photograph, and I'm saying that your whole testimony was one which was emotionally charged."

"My mother was a lawyer and there is a word in French for that," she said, disclosing at last how she had acquired her court room confidence. "You are judging my intention. You have got no right to do that. I can take you to court for doing that to me. What I said was true. That is what I feel about you."

"Well, feel free to do so, Mrs. Souter. The point is, that was exactly your intention. I am telling you that you delivered a testimony here which was emotionally charged and was inaccurate."

"I can take you to court for that, according to French law."

"Well, we happen to be in Pretoria at the moment," he said, looking as though he was congratulating himself on this advocate-like reply.

Chapter 18

Ailing Advocate's Secret

There was another postponement. Four months later, the inquiry began again with the ailing Goldblum telling the Committee that the condition of his health remained the same, however the Defense would now be conducted by his co-counsel, Advocate Nadine Havenga, so that the proceedings would not be interrupted in the future by his physical problems. As things turned out, Havenga's entry appeared to be another one of Lieberthal's delaying tactics. She was allowed to object to one thing after another.

First of all, there was a long discussion about the fact that the hearing, at that time, had been set down for two weeks and an adjournment was necessary because she would only be available to defend Lieberthal for the first week. The Committee threw that one out, ruling that Lieberthal had agreed to the new time frame, although "he now does not recall that," the Chairman remarked. Lieberthal was told to make the best of it.

Dr. Barnard had hardly said, "So we'll continue now," when it became clear that the Defense was once again getting VIP treatment. The hearing was transformed into a John Grisham-like courtroom drama, where a Defense attorney suddenly protests: "this is a trial by ambush," when the prosecution announced it was calling a surprise witness. Havenga used virtually the same description to describe Berger's intention to call witnesses he had previously said would not be coming. After being allowed to argue this point with Berger for hours, she eventually conceded that they could be called. Lieberthal's side had scored another time wasting goal.

Before this chapter was over, Berger said, "It is odd that initially there was an objection on the basis that we were not calling the patients to testify, and now there is an objection that we are calling them. It is a trite principle in law that one cannot approbate and reprobate or, as it is colloquially put, one cannot blow hot and cold at the same time."

Havenga solved the mystery as to why Goldblum was working for nothing. "From what I understand, Dr. Lieberthal has performed operations on my learned friend Mr. Goldblum, also on a pro amico basis. So there is this measure of tit for tat; there is a friendship. I owe Dr. Lieberthal no such allegiance, nor does any other counsel. We want our fees."

Goldblum died three years after the hearing ended and I asked his widow what she thought of the treatment her husband received from Lieberthal. "*Ag*, you know what, they had a very different relationship. I would rather not get involved in it, thank you," was her loaded reply that conjured up all kinds of possibilities.

Cotterell, the Rosebank Clinic manager when Lieberthal was there, said to me, "Lieberthal has an advocate, Goldblum. You investigate him. I think he's part of the problem. Goldblum was in our ICU at one stage while I was there and somebody caustically remarked he's getting Pethidine in large doses. I think he was addicted to this drug, which Lieberthal was supplying."

The inquiry was running rudderless most of the time, with Lieberthal's team being allowed complete freedom to tack backwards and forwards, endlessly. This only added to the cost of the hearing, which must have been a legal eagle's dream.

I shuddered to think what any of his aggrieved patients must have thought of the way the proceedings were being conducted; so much in the doctor's favor. There was nobody strong enough on the Committee's side to put a stop to Lieberthal's crafty manipulation because they were haunted by the fear that they might be accused of not being fair to the unfortunate media-persecuted surgeon.

On one of the few occasions that there was any criticism of the way the inquiry was going, Strauss said, "Must we again postpone this matter? It has a long history of postponements, fairly lengthy ones. Sooner or later, this matter must come to an end, hopefully. It cannot carry on indefinitely. A variety of interests are at stake here. Last, but not least, I would say, actually the foremost interest is that of the complainants. They are entitled to come and tell this Committee what their complaints are all about."

Poor, hurting Mrs. Lawson, who Dr. Craig described as having, "intractable back pain for which I know of no orthopedic treatment," had now been waiting for two days to tell her story while those at the inquiry waffled on with absolutely no regard for the agony she might have been in. Nobody appeared to consider that she was not the average, normal, healthy witness; otherwise, she would not have been there.

The Committee overruled all Havenga's main objections. With an hour to go in the day, she asked for another recess to "take instructions" from her client.

Perplexed, Berger said, "I am not quite sure what that means because Mrs. Lawson has not given evidence yet."

She would have to wait a lot longer if Havenga had her way. "Mr. Chairman, with regard to your response to what I had placed on record previously with regards to the remarks made by yourself, my instructions are that my client did not interpret this as a slight against myself. He interpreted the comment and the subsequent laughter as a clear indication of the lack of impartiality of the tribunal. And that there was a clear indication that the tribunal had already decided the outcome of the application even before my reply, to his detriment. Now, having said that, my client wishes to consider his position in this regard."

She was referring to the Chairman's monumental boo-boo during a lunch break. She and Lieberthal overheard him saying to Professor Strauss, "*Dit is maar "n desperate poging van haar* (it was a desperate attempt of hers)".

After hedging for a while, she eventually said they wanted to "possibly take this tribunal on review," or to "make a recusal application."

The ball was tossed to Berger as the game continued with nobody seemingly able to make a decisive shot. He said there was no basis for a review at that stage.

The next morning, Havenga opened by saying, "I wish to bring an application for recusal of the Committee for the reasons that this tribunal is clearly biased against my client. My client's perception is that it does not matter what he does, the Committee has already made up its mind."

Point scoring went on and on once again, back and forth across the net as if they were trying to get into the Guinness Book of Records, with more and more decided cases thrown in.

Berger's view was that the application had "no merit whatsoever". It was just another "desperate attempt by Lieberthal to prevent the finalization of this matter". When the application was refused, Havenga brought another one. She asked for time to consider taking the Committee's decision on review to the High Court.

In opposing this, Berger referred to the case of Dr. Illes versus the Health Profession Council. Illes" radiological practice had been caught giving kickbacks to specialists for sending them patients. There had been a disciplinary inquiry similar to the Lieberthal one, which had gone on for many months. Illes applied to the High Court to have the proceedings adjourned. What that involved, Berger said, was "in essence" the same as the one Havenga was now proposing.

In dismissing the Illes application, Judge Botha said that the "well known approach" was that a court should be loath to interfere in pending proceedings in another court unless it was clear that a grave injustice would be done. He found no evidence of this. Nothing was done in nine months when all that Illes was complaining about could have been addressed. Lieberthal was evidently not the only doctor who gave the HPC the run around.

"As was said in the Illes case," Burger continued. "It would be unfair to complainants, who have already testified, it would be unfair to the patients who still have to testify, it would be unfair to the prosecution that has to organize and bear substantial costs for these proceedings, if they were simply to be adjourned so that Dr. Lieberthal could, at his leisure, approach the High Court on review. There is a duty on the Health Professions Council to ensure that these proceedings are brought to a conclusion sooner, rather than later."

Lunch was taken, and Mrs. Lawson was still being kept waiting. Afterwards, the Committee refused a postponement for Lieberthal to make his High Court application. It would have taken six months or a year before this could be heard.

That was one defeat too many for the defiant surgeon. Havenga reacted by saying, "Thank you Mr. Chairman, members of the tribunal, Professor Strauss, we will now excuse ourselves. Thank you." Lieberthal stomped out in a huff with his legal team. He was unaccustomed to not being able to manipulate events in his favor.

Somewhat taken aback by this turn of events, the Chairman once again asked Professor Strauss for guidance. "Mr. Chairman, my advice is that, as the accused has decided not to be present at the hearing, from now on the validity of the proceedings will not be affected. They can carry on in the absence of the Defense, as relatively frequently happens in inquiries of this nature."

The "bend over backwards to help Lieberthal"-theme continued even after he had walked out as the Professor commented, "In the circumstances, I would advise that the panel may perhaps be somewhat more active in putting questions to witnesses, than otherwise would be the case, for the sake of being absolutely fair. This is because of the absence of counsel to cross-examine on behalf of the Defense."

Berger at last called Martha Hendrina Willemina Lawson to give evidence.

There was a long list of heart-rending stories resulting from Lieberthal's noxious treatment, but Lawson's turned out to be one of the most harrowing. He had left behind a shell of a woman who had aged well beyond her 52 years. She needed a walking stick for support.

The surgeon had robbed her of all self-esteem, so much so that she related her tale in a faltering voice that was almost a whisper. On several occasions, it was necessary to ask her to speak up.

Her distressing back history began early. At 15, she injured her spine when the school bus overturned. "When my mum came and fetched me," she told Berger, "she said, 'Why can my child not walk?' I could not put one foot in front of the other. I could only move sideways." Physiotherapy over a period of two years enabled her to walk properly unassisted.

After she gave birth to two daughters and a son and entered her forties, she started experiencing more and more lower back pain. What was perhaps the biggest tragedy in her turbulent life, especially from a mother's point of view, was that her son was brain damaged after an epileptic fit when he was three. At 13, when he became too big for her to look after, he was put into Avril Elizabeth House.

She saw Lieberthal in February 1998, and after looking at her x-rays, he told her that he would have to do a fusion, as she had broken her neck at some stage. "I did not know that I had ever had that, but I presume if you have broken your neck, you got quite severe problems," she told Berger.

Lieberthal also diagnosed a tumor at the back of her spine.

"I took his word that I had a tumor in my spine," she continued, "because I do not know x-rays or anything. I was shocked." This former Absa Bank personnel department employee then had the first of four operations, from which she had never recovered, and Lieberthal still wanted to do another one.

She didn't go back to him because "the same operation, a fusion at L3, 4 and 5 that he wanted to do in 2002, was what he did in 1998." At one stage, she became very ill because of an allergic reaction to the Valeron Lieberthal put her on over a period of three months. She had a bad bout of depression.

Crying, she explained that, in January 1999, "I was in terrible… at that time I was very, very suicidal and depressed. I actually, went to my boss the one morning, and I said to him, 'I feel worthless', because I…. You know, I realize that I am going to lose my job."

Trying to pacify her, Berger said, "It's alright, take your time."

"And with the fact that I cannot bring my son home any more either," she added with the tears running down her cheeks.

The Chairman wanted to adjourn to allow her to "compose herself", but Lawson said she was "fine", although this hardly seemed to be the case.

Initially, she had been advised by her psychologist that, because of her "emotional state", it would not be good for her health to testify. However, she told the Committee, "If Dr. Lieberthal did something that he was not supposed to do, I have forgiven him. This is why I could come here and testify today: to help to stop him doing wrong to anybody else if he has done wrong, because I know the pain that I endured, and I'm sure that everybody who testified knew the way their lives had changed. The reason why I am testifying is not to get anything out of this. I just want justice done."

It looked as though she would get her way when Professor Lukhele's opinion was taken into account. His findings painted a dismal picture of an incompetent surgeon who had harmed his patient by doing one unnecessary operation after another.

Lieberthal's handiwork had left Maria Whitaker in such a bad way that she was bedridden at her home in Port Elizabeth when the inquiry took place. She died not long afterwards, having had to endure a pain level for years that had almost gone off the scale.

Maria had five lumbar back operations by Lieberthal before she moved from Johannesburg to Port Elizabeth to be near her sisters. The first one was in January 1999 when she was aged 58. She came round so full of drugs that had been prescribed that she fell out of bed. That didn't say much for the standard of nursing care, let alone what Lieberthal was doing to her.

"She snapped the one vertebra right off," her husband Eldred told me.

If only she had listened to orthopedic surgeon Bruce Bailie at Alberton. She saw him a year earlier when she first began suffering from pains in her buttocks. He did not think an operation was advisable. She was subsequently sent to Lieberthal by Dr. H. Khoury, her GP in Rosettenville.

As she could not come to Pretoria, Dr. Armaud Morkel, a neurosurgeon at the Queen Acres Hospital in Port Elizabeth, gave evidence because he had been managing her pain. "I expect rehabilitation not to be successful," he told Berger. "I have to conclude that she is probably going to suffer from pain permanently."

He mentioned a whole basket full of drugs she had been in an attempt to control her chronic pain, which was still "utterly severe." It remained rated by her as high as eight out of ten. "She is at present on Morphine Sulphate tablets, which I am lucky to say are having a relatively beneficial effect on her pain."

Her auditor husband was disillusioned by the Medical Council for not calling him to give evidence about how Lieberthal instructed him to give his wife Pethidine injections at home. "That was a major problem for me because they kicked that charge out," he told me. "I could have got evidence from the pharmacist about all the prescriptions Dr. Lieberthal gave me. But I was never called, and they made a decision without referring to me."

Visagie had been living in Windhoek, having left Johannesburg three years earlier. This 50-year-old diamond polisher was operated on by Lieberthal on three occasions. The first operation was in June 1999 and the last one was in January 2001. He too was initially admitted in a hurry after being told that a piece of broken vertebra was causing pressure on the nerve.

The operation transformed him into a badly made tin toy soldier. When he was walking, he could hear a "cluck, cluck, cluck" noise in his back. "It was terrible sounding," he said. He heard this after the first operation. It was not very loud then. After his check-up it got worse and his back started hurting again so he went back to Lieberthal and more x-rays were taken. "He said to me, sorry to say, but he has to operate again. The cluck, cluck noise is coming from one of the screws that had come loose."

The benefits of the operation that followed in November 1999 did not last long. In January the following year, Lieberthal told him the screws had come loose again because of his smoking and being overweight.

In a depressed state, he saw Dr. Craig for a second opinion. Before he went, he deleted Lieberthal's name from his x-ray records. Asked by the Chairman why he had done this, he said, "There are certain doctors who protect each other and I did not want Dr. Craig to see who had been operating on me, because they might be colleagues." Craig was not fooled. "After he examined me, he said, 'Dr. Wynne Lieberthal operated on you'. I asked him how does he know and he said he knows his work. Now, what he meant by that, I do not know."

Craig had advised him to live with the pain and not have any further operations. But it became so unbearable that he went back to Lieberthal for a third operation because no other doctors would touch him.

The evidence Professor Mkhize gave upheld everything in the charge sheet, and some of his uncomplimentary comments made Lieberthal's case look more hopeless than ever.

It was well documented that the success of spine operations decreases with every repeat operation, he told the Committee. "With the third operation, it is no more than thirty percent with the success rate for subsequent ones even less." It was also 'unethical' to give a 'high risk treatment to a patient when the benefits do not outweigh the risk'.

In the early part of the inquiry, Goldblum had tried to discredit the Professor's role as an expert witness because he had not examined any of the complainants. This was not necessary, Mkhize retorted, because if he was to examine them he would only be able to establish the condition they were in long after the events complained of.

"Do you believe, sir, that an expert opinion can be formulated purely on written submissions and radiological investigations?" Goldblum put to him.

"It's pretty sound practice. The x-rays are objective. They cannot fool you. And secondly, the colleague's clinic notes are there, and thirdly the colleague's response, which was written through you, was there and then the complainants had various operation reports."

"The Defense contends, Professor that you appear to be painting the worst possible scenario pertaining to my client."

Mkhize's justification was that he was trying to be as scientific and objective as possible, both for Goldblum's client and the complainants. "That is the function of an expert witness. There are no personal feelings involved."

"I accept that, but I do not believe it has been done in this forum," was Goldblum's parting shot.

At the end of the evidence presented by Advocate Berger, he ripped into the surgeon in very disparaging terms. "Our submission is that it is patently clear that Dr. Lieberthal has conducted himself in an improper, disgraceful, dishonorable and unworthy manner. We say he failed to address problems that could, and should, have been addressed if he had exercised the care and skill that is reasonably expected of a competent spine surgeon.

"There are so many examples where the job is either incomplete or not properly done, involving operating in the wrong place; misplacing screws and having them come loose. In some instances, they are so badly misplaced that this causes problems by impinging onto nerves, necessitating further operations. From this, one gets a picture of a surgeon who is intent on doing as many operations as he possibly can, regardless of whether those operations are indicated or necessary, and without ensuring that he takes the time that is needed to conduct the operations properly.

"It appears to us that the explanation for all these rushed operations was financial. If Dr. Lieberthal had given evidence, I would have put that to him to see what his explanation was. But in the absence of him giving evidence, we cannot think of another inference which would explain all these mistakes.

"I think one can safely exclude incompetence as a reason for all the problems which are apparent from the evidence. That leaves reckless behavior, reckless in the sense of how the operations were carried out. In some instances, it was deliberate when he told Broda that she had a possible underlying cancerous tumor when there was no cancer, and that Lawson required urgent surgery to remove a tumor when he never removed one. He instills fear in a patient to get them to agree to urgent surgery. That is worse than recklessness."

Concluding the case for the Council, Berger said, "So we submit, Mr. Chairperson and members of the Committee that Dr. Lieberthal ought to be found guilty on all the charges, one through to seven."

A few months later, in July 2004, the Committee announced its decision. The case had taken more than a year to be finalized. The verdict was guilty, guilty, guilty, seven times over. It found that Lieberthal's professional conduct fell short of what was reasonably required of an orthopedic surgeon who does spinal surgery.

In sentencing Lieberthal to be struck off the register, Dr. Barnard said, "We are of the opinion that the seven charges against Lieberthal are of a serious nature. Many of his patients have sustained permanent bodily harm as a result of his actions and will probably suffer from pain for the rest of their lives."

In the layperson's world, that would be called "grievous bodily harm" and it would undoubtedly have attracted a stiff prison sentence if done on the kind of scale that Lieberthal did it.

Danny Berger had asked for a heavy sentence to be imposed and, in doing so, he pointed out that Lieberthal had never apologized and nor had he admitted that he had ever made a mistake. "Instead, he adopted the attitude of having done nothing wrong. This is the most frightening aspect of the case. We cannot allow a doctor who does not admit he is wrong to continue to practice."

A peculiar aspect of the penalty the Council imposed was that it gave no length of time for Lieberthal's suspension.

The medical profession breathed a sigh of relief. With its most notorious butcher confined to the wilderness, it could once more sink back into obscurity, which was just the way it liked it. At least, that's what everybody thought.

Anybody who believed our specialist would be spending his time sitting around a swimming pool sipping a glass of wine, or whatever his tipple happened to be, was very much mistaken. He was too ingenious for that.

Just under two years after Lieberthal was struck off, he was back in the news with The Star proclaiming, "Disgraced SA surgeon probed by Irish army."

Unfazed by the decision to prevent him practicing in South Africa, Lieberthal got a job as a GP within months of being deregistered. He signed a lucrative one-year contract with the Irish Defense Force to treat the troops in its peacekeeping force in Liberia, North Africa.

It was only after he had completed his assignment in Monrovia and returned to South Africa that the scandal riddled-doctor's name was raised in none other than the Irish Parliament or D`ail. His notoriety had gone international and was considered serious enough to be discussed by that country's Minister of Defense.

Medical Solutions of Chessington in Surrey, the employment agency in England that had got the contract to supply doctors for the Irish army, had slipped up badly. Checks, if any, that had been made into Lieberthal's background, missed the vital fact that he had been banned from practicing in his home country. He must have been very amused at how careless people can be, even when it's their job to sift through employment applications to make sure their clients get no unpleasant surprises.

Speaking in the D`ail, a contrite Willie O'Dea, the Minister of Defense, said, "I share the Deputy's concern that this situation should have arisen. My first priority in dealing with this is the welfare of the troops who were attended to by this man. To that end, the Director of the Medical Corps has contacted each person who had served in Liberia during the period in question, alerting them to the situation. There appeared to be nothing whatsoever untoward in the CV supplied in respect of Dr. Lieberthal."

Lieberthal was initially appointed for a three-month period from December 2004 and was then retained in Liberia until December 2005, when the overall contract with Medicare Solutions expired. He provided medical care to the Irish troops and a small contingent from Sweden, largely on a routine general practitioner level.

Medicare Solutions had the contract from June 2004. It was renewed in March 2005 at E2 630 per doctor per week and ended when the Defense Force was able to provide its own doctors from the Medical Corps.

Assuming that Lieberthal had earned, say, E2 000 per week, or E104 000 for the 52 weeks he was in the Army, the rand equivalent at the exchange rate of approximately R8 to the euro would have been close to a million rand. In addition, his living expenses would no doubt have been provided by the army while he was in Liberia.

"I am extremely concerned as to how this situation arose and I will ensure that all necessary steps are taken to avoid any possible repetition," O'Dea assured Parliament. Legal advice was being obtained about the performance of the recruitment agency. The requirement to pursue Irish Medical Council registration was included in the contract with the agency. Lieberthal had applied for this, but never obtained it.

"The delay in identifying this failure will form part of the report on the situation," said O'Dea. "While the safeguards will be reviewed along with the performance of the agency, it should be pointed out that, in the first instance, the person himself should not have commenced work, based on falsehoods."

Captain Feargal Purcell at the Defense Force's Press Office told me that they were made aware that Lieberthal had been struck off by one of their own members. There had been no complaints to the hotline that had been set up from any of the troops who had been treated by Lieberthal. The report that was completed into the investigation would not be made public. "Suffice to say, we are satisfied that the failure was at the initial recruitment stage, which was not carried out by the Defense Forces."

Despite this huge, well-publicized indictment of his honesty, while he was under suspension, all those who suffered because of Lieberthal's actions reckoned without the Health Profession Council's incredible ability to forgive, no matter how appalling the record of this doctor might have been. Maimed and paralyzed patients counted for little in their eyes when balanced against getting the much-needed skills of an orthopedic surgeon back into the operating theater.

Chapter 19

Legal Vultures

All the publicity soon attracted the legal vultures. They flew in from all directions to feast on Lieberthal's rotten cases. There were certainly rich pickings to be had, as the funds available from his malpractice insurers were virtually limitless. The attorneys did not have to worry about whether the doctor himself had the means to meet their massive demands.

Mervyn Joseph of Joseph's Incorporated was probably the most successful. He specialized in medical malpractice and personal injury claims. He sued Lieberthal for the following amounts on behalf of various clients: R6 103 087 (Mariskca du Plessis); R3 747 226 (Sean Cooper); R3 256 049 (Jennifer Musgrove) and R2 700 000 (Piet Strauss), making a total of R15 806 362.

Other attorneys, who appeared to have been a bit slow in leaving their plush offices to soar over the landscape, also got some of the action. Stephen Flowers of Munro, Flowers and Vermaak, got a R2 200 000 payment for his client, Jacqui Baleta. Mervyn Gross of Bloch Gross and Associates picked up some crumbs when he claimed R863 966 on behalf of Yossi Donino. There may have been others that I was unable to find.

Settlements were reached in all the cases, sometimes for less than the amounts demanded, effectively admitting that Lieberthal was guilty as hell.

I heard that the Medical Protection Society had been forced to put up its premiums for doctors because of all the money it had to fork out for Lieberthal's claims, but this was not the case, John Middleton, the Membership Adviser, assured me. He refused to divulge how much Lieberthal had cost the Society, or whether it would ever cover him again on the grounds that this was "confidential".

The attorneys for the claimants took their instructions on a contingency basis at a fee of around 25 percent of the amounts recovered after deducting costs for medico-legal reports. The doctor provided a veritable mint for these birds that thrive on the misfortunes of others, but still have a role to play in cleaning up the veldt.

For their clients, all the money in the world could not prevent most of them from continuing a life of misery which, in at least one case, did not last very long. There were other cases where Lieberthal's patients died soon after he had treated them, but they had not brought actions for damages against him.

Sadly, Sean Cooper, who detonated the explosion of publicity, did not live to benefit from the money that was paid in his case, not that it could have done much to improve his health. He died aged 33 in his sleep in May 2006, just three and a half months after the birth of his daughter, Unter, who was his first child. This was before his malpractice action was finalized. His young wife, Tanya, continued with the case as executor of his estate. By that time, she had moved from Johannesburg and was living with her parents in Durban.

Psychiatrist Dr. David Shevel, who years earlier had reported on Lieberthal for the purposes of one of his insurance claims, was on the opposite side this time. Cooper told him that, while in hospital, he was hearing voices and seeing apparitions. "At that stage, he was high on doses of analgesic medication and he believes he was even on Pethidine 100 mgs up to eight times a day."

After he left hospital, he had panic attacks, sometimes every half an hour. He had palpitations; he hyperventilated and suffered from nausea, dizziness, and increased perspiration. "During a panic attack, Mr. Cooper is concerned that he is losing control and that he is having a heart attack," Shevel wrote. "When asked why he feels worthless, he answered, 'Because of what I was and what I am now. I was a supreme athlete and a good businessman. Now I'm a waste of a body, doing really badly.'

"He became addicted to the drugs Lieberthal gave him while he was in hospital," his wife told me. At her wit's end as to how to cope with him, she served him with divorce papers at one stage. She later put the case on hold.

When he was seen by Shevel in November 2004, he was still suffering from chronic pain, and Dr. Edeling predicted he could not expect any improvement as his back was likely to further deteriorate requiring major salvage, lumbar surgery. With such a bleak future, he may well have chosen to deliberately end his life by taking an overdose of one of the drugs he was prescribed. Alternatively, he could have accidentally taken too many.

As his death was an unnatural one, an inquest had to be held. But the state tended to move depressingly slowly in cases like this. More than a year after his death, no inquest had been held. It could not even begin without the autopsy results from the state pathologist, which were not yet available. Tanya very much wanted to clear up the mystery of exactly what caused his death. If it could be pinned on the treatment he got from Lieberthal, she intended suing him for an additional amount.

Jennifer Musgrove was a 35-year-old divorced, single mother of two in September 2002, when she consulted Lieberthal for lower back pain. He operated and did a fusion.

Her initial experience was very similar to Mariskca du Plessis" when she returned from surgery. She couldn't move her legs. During the next two days, she continued to complain that she had no sensation from the waist down. On the fourth day, Lieberthal did his notorious disappearing act. He left for overseas, leaving Musgrove in the care of his locum, Dr. Golding.

Fortunately for her, Dr. Golding turned out to be a vast improvement on the departing surgeon. He immediately arranged for an MRI scan, and Dr. Hoffmann was asked to examine her. He concluded she had a blood clot next to her spinal cord and that urgent surgery was needed to remove it. He operated and took out the clot.

The feeling in her legs began to return and when she was discharged from hospital about a month after her first operation, she was able to walk with crutches and splints on her legs. She will have to use these splints for the rest of her life.

In her claim, she accused Lieberthal of "failing to treat or prevent" the complication she suffered when "by the exercise of reasonable skill, care and diligence expected of a specialist orthopedic surgeon, he could and should have done so."

Jenny, an internal saleswoman before she was disabled, did not want to go over her harrowing experience with Lieberthal when I spoke to her. However, some years earlier she told You magazine that before her operation she saw some large screws that had been removed from a fellow patient in her ward.

"I asked Dr. Lieberthal if he was going to use similar screws in my back and he assured me he would only use bond," she told the magazine. Inevitably, when she was given her post-operative x-rays, they showed screws in her spine, all six of them.

Lieberthal relied on that patient confidentiality cop-out when You magazine spoke to him. "I can't comment further on her case without her permission. The patient knew what needed to be done and signed a consent form."

It was not only his back that was troubling Piet Strauss when I saw him in his rather ordinary house close to an industrial area in Alberton. He was an extremely unhappy man. Money certainly had not brought him happiness. An Afrikaner, he spoke good English with a few Afrikaans words thrown in from time to time.

A short, balding man close to 60, he told me very emotionally, "I'm going to tell you now. The day I went to collect my check, my lawyer told me. 'I hope you…'" He broke off as his eyes began to glisten. It was obvious he didn't want me to see him break down. He was having a battle containing the hurt that was welling up behind those eyes of his. Severe ongoing back pain would make even grown men cry quite easily. In his case, he had considerable emotional stress, as well.

"'You and your wife are okay'," he continued relating what he had been told. "'Because why, she can take you to the cleaners.' And she's doing that, *meneer*. I'm busy with the divorce case now."

His wife, Erina, was a human resources manager at a steel company where she had worked for 16 years. They had been married for almost 30 years and had two children in their twenties.

"What does she say the problem is in your marriage?" I asked.

"I don't know *meneer*. It all started in December 2005. A month after I got my money from Lieberthal, she started with this shit, so that money gave me more heartache and pain than the operation."

He went into the kitchen and returned to the lounge with two cups of tea, one of which he put on the table in front of me. By this time, he was more composed.

"How many operations did Dr. Lieberthal do on you?" I asked.

"One main one, but when he did that, he operated on my neck and my back under the same anesthetic."

In the letter of complaint that the three surgeons had sent to the Health Professions Council, they deplored this kind of multiple surgery, done under the same anesthetic as it was "not an internationally recognized surgical practice," but that did not stop Lieberthal doing it on several other patients, besides Strauss.

In the 1970s, Strauss had woken up one morning with a stiff neck and, after his doctor had done some manipulation in hospital, he had no further problems until 1996. Then, while working as a store's manager at a refrigeration company, he began to get pins and needles in his feet at night. His GP sent him to Dr. Snyckers, who diagnosed a problem in his neck. No operation was considered necessary. His symptoms continued, so in 2002, he decided to do something more positive about them.

Lieberthal had been recommended to him by Jenny de Wet, the wife of the *dominee* at his local Nederduitsch Gereformeerde church. "She thought he was the 'best surgeon in the country' after he operated on her neck," he said.

Strauss' first appointment was cancelled because Lieberthal had broken his arm while weight lifting. When he finally saw him, he was impressed by the doctor's "beautiful" office. "*Jirre* man, he was so interested in my case. What a nice guy. He sent me over the road to the Rosebank Clinic to have x-rays and when I brought them back he said, 'Jesus *meneer*, you've got a problem. A piece of bone from one of the vertebra in your neck has broken off and is lying between the main artery and the main nerve'. He showed me on the x-ray."

"Could you see something?" I asked.

"Well, I'm no expert. There was something. I believed him. He said, 'If you fell, or you whip lashed your neck in a car accident, I guarantee you will be paralyzed. This is urgent. I must operate on you within the next week. If not, I'm telling you now, go and buy yourself an electric wheel chair because you'll be paralyzed.' Hell, I got a big *skrik, jees*."

Strauss had never had a back problem. He did his own gardening and was a keen fisherman. Two months before he saw Lieberthal, he went on holiday down to the coast with his caravan. "I was fishing the whole three weeks, jumping from rock to rock and going into the sea. We even went out with the ski boat deep sea fishing. Now a man with a back problem can't do that."

"So you only went to see him because of this tingling in your feet?"

"*Ja*, that's all. But when he told me about this bit of bone in my neck, he said, 'You've also got lower back problems. While we are doing this operation, let's do your back at the same time, otherwise you'll be back here within the next two or three years. Let's *sommer* do it once.' So I told him, 'Oh hell let's do it then.'"

Lieberthal also gave him a weird "guarantee" that after the operation he would have "an erection like he had never had before." This was in spite of the fact that Strauss had not complained about any problem in that area.

Concerned about the open plastic cast his surgeon had on his arm, Strauss said to him, "Can't my operation wait until your arm has healed?" Lieberthal replied, "No, this is an emergency. Don't worry about my arm. I've already done eight operations, very successfully."

Strauss remembered asking about Lieberthal's success rate. "I was told that, apart from one or two septic wounds, it was 99.9 percent. He gave me no time to change my mind. After I saw him on the Monday, he operated the following Wednesday.

"On the morning before the operation he didn't come to see me in the ward," Piet said, wiping his nose with a tissue as his eyes began to water again. "Not even the anesthetist came to see me. *Jirre*, I was upset, *jong*. While they were pushing me into the theatre, I was crying. I just wanted to get off the trolley. The anesthetist then walked over to me and said, 'I was supposed to come and see you in the ward.'"

"Who was he, Patterson?" I asked.

"Patterson, *ja*. He asked me a few questions and said, 'Don't worry we'll sort you out.'"

"What did he ask you?"

"If I've got high blood pressure or diabetes. I can't remember everything. It only took a couple of seconds because I was going into theatre."

Strauss went back to see Lieberthal two weeks after the operation because of a swelling at the site of the wound in his back. It was caused by internal bleeding, Lieberthal said, and he drained it with a syringe. "He didn't want to see me," Piet said. "When I walked into his consulting room, he didn't invite me to sit down. At that stage, I was in terrible pain."

"So after the operation his attitude changed completely, did it?" I asked.

"Completely, completely. He was a different person. He was actually aggressive; very nasty to me. At one stage, he even told me 'There's nothing wrong with you'. But I was still a lamppost. I couldn't bend, I couldn't walk and, according to him, he was satisfied with my progress. That's when I saw this person is a bloody arsehole, man."

Within a week of the lump in his back being drained, it got even bigger so

Lieberthal decided to readmit him for an operation to stop the bleeding. In the waiting area, when he was about to go into theatre, he saw Patterson.

"That's when he said to me, 'I was wondering when we were going to see you again'. Then he turned around and walked away. I was so full of pain I didn't think much about it at the time."

Every time he consulted Lieberthal after the initial operation, he was sent for more x-rays. "There were screws and bars in my spine, when he told me he was not going to use these."

His operation cost R127 000, most of it paid for by his medical aid, although he still had to pay some of this himself. He was given a "whole lot of pills" to take home. "Jesus, I was so tranquilized it was not true. I couldn't see. I couldn't think. I was like a bloody drunk, lying in bed, sick to my stomach. My wife tried to phone him. To begin with, she couldn't get hold of him. Eventually, when she did speak to him, he said throw those pills away. They cost me R1 200 which I had to pay myself."

As he was still suffering after the bleeding had stopped, Lieberthal told him to exercise in a swimming pool. As this did not help, he returned to his GP, who sent him to Dr. Bruce Bailie at the Union Hospital. He was the same orthopedic surgeon who advised Maria Whitaker not to have surgery before Lieberthal did five lumbar spine operations on her.

"When he looked at my x-rays he said, 'This is the biggest *kak* job I've ever seen in my life. You must sue this oke.' I imagined something happened in the past between Bailie and Lieberthal because Bailie knew this guy. He actually told me Lieberthal was a drug addict. 'You must report him to the Medical Council,' he said. 'If you're not going to do it, I'll do it on your behalf.'

"So I sent them a letter. They said they've investigated my complaint, and they found nothing wrong."

That was so characteristic of the way the Council dismissed cases despite strong evidence to support a disciplinary hearing inquiry. It must have been overwhelming if Strauss was able to get the payout he received.

Dr. Marus, who prepared a medico-legal report for Strauss" case, concluded there was no necessity to operate on either Strauss's neck or his back. To cap it all, he revealed that the fusion in Piet's back had failed and he had broken metal rods in that area.

After reading Mariskca du Plessis' story in The Star, Strauss visited her, and her mother told him about Mervyn Joseph. "I phoned him and asked him to help me out," he told me. "I went to his office the next day, and he said, 'You've got a very good case. I'll take it. Sign here.'

"Mervyn phoned me and said he managed to get R2.7 million. I ended up with around R1.2-million after Mervyn's fees and other deductions. In total, I saw 14 specialists in connection with this case, eight or nine from our side and the rest from the opposition."

Describing his condition when I saw him five years after Lieberthal had operated on him, he said, "While I'm sitting here, it feels like I've got two solid balls in my back, as big as cricket balls. After the operation, I had a buzzing sound in my ears. I went from one ENT specialist to the other, but nobody could cure it. My hearing is stuffed, my bowel is stuffed and my manhood is stuffed. Every night, I must take a sleeping tablet, otherwise I hear this buzzing sound when everything is quiet."

The way he moved, I could see his back was giving him a lot of pain.

When the operation was done, he had been employed for eight years by Reco Refrigeration in Johannesburg as its central warehouse controller, where there was R18-million worth of equipment. He had spent most of his time in the warehouse, moving about, checking stock.

"They treated me very badly," he said. "After the operation, I was off work for three months. When I went back, I worked for a year in terrible pain."

His efforts to continue working were evidently not appreciated by his firm. He was charged at a disciplinary inquiry with exceeding his sick leave by 39 days. "They found me guilty of misconduct, or whatever you call it. I was referred to Dr. George Zwonnikoff, who is a neurosurgeon. Luckily he told them, 'This man is suffering, board the guy.'"

"What did he say when he looked at your x-rays?" I wanted to know.

"He said he can't find anything wrong with the procedure, but the operation was unnecessary."

"Does it still mean you get a pension?"

"*Ja*, luckily I'm getting 75% of my salary. I had a hell of a fight. They brought in people from the CCMA to handle my case and I can tell you they really grilled me. If it wasn't for Dr. Zwonnikoff, I was stuffed for the rest of my life with no pension. That R1.2-million doesn't last a lifetime."

"On what grounds were they trying to get out of paying you?"

"They thought, and they still think, I'm not really that bad."

"In other words, they thought you were a malingerer."

"*Ja*, that's the word. That's why every year I must go and see a doctor for a checkup and a report."

Having read a report about his successful action against Lieberthal in The Star, Pam Bekink phoned him. "I visited her and she can hardly walk, hey," he said. "When I left I was crying, *meneer*. I don't know if she's still alive. She also phoned this Du Plessis family. I think she phoned us because she thought we could give her some money. Nobody wants to help her. She's in dire straits. But I couldn't support her. I had my son and daughter who were at varsity. I gave her some money, 100 bucks here and there, but that's all I could do."

I left Strauss with nothing pleasant to look forward to except a constant, painful reminder of Dr. Lieberthal. Dr. Marus had a gloomy prediction for his neck and back. "He will have to undergo further lumbar surgery to repair the non-union. It is likely that he will have ongoing, chronic mechanical neck and lumbar symptoms with secondary effects of chronic pain on his psyche.

Chapter 20

Unkindest Cut Of All

As if Jacqui Baleta didn't have enough to contend with. It had happened a little over a week before I saw her, and she still had the "shakes" when she talked about it. Her Lieberthal experience had temporarily taken a back seat.

A traumatic event like this would take most people years to adjust to. Even then, it would remain menacingly in their subconscious, ready to jolt them back to reality at the slightest provocation.

The forty-one-year-old mother of two and her partner, Larry Hendriks, were asleep in one of the two upstairs bedrooms of their spacious house in Oakdene in the southern part of Johannesburg. Her fifteen-year-old daughter Annastazia, Stassy for short, was also in the land of nod in the bedroom next door.

Outside, the foul night was tailor made for evil deeds. A typical Highveld summer storm was raging. Bright flashes were darting through the clouds that rumbled and crashed as heavy rain poured from them, blotting out all other sounds. This was the perfect cover, just what the predators needed. They were on the prowl, like hungry panthers, with their black bodies glistening as the water ran off them and the shining objects in their hands.

It was a chilling sight, had anybody been there to see them. They had chosen well. Nobody else was likely to be out in that weather, two hours past midnight. They were just like thousands of others who were busy terrorizing an entire nation on nights like this and even in broad daylight.

"Larry sleeps like the dead, so he thought he was dreaming at first," Jacqui told me. The dream of this forty-five-year-old electrician turned into a real life nightmare, as scary as any you could think of.

Describing what happened, Baleta said, "The two of us suddenly realized we had two black men in the bedroom determined to kill us. They were each wielding claw hammers. Larry, who used to be a bodybuilder, put both of them down and each time one went down, the other one would come back at him."

While the fight raged on, one of the intruders broke away and went to Stassy's room, just as she was opening the door to see what was happening.

"The two of them got into a scuffle but, thank goodness, Stassy had no serious injuries, just a few bruises," said Baleta. "Of course, she has been mentally scarred for life."

Somehow, Hendriks managed to bundle his two assailants down the stairs. There had been a third black man stealing various things on the ground floor, and the three of them were debating whether to rush up the stairs. "Larry kept shouting to Stassy and I, 'Phone the cops, phone the cops'. The men were telling us to keep quiet and one of them said they had a gun. I might not be speaking to you now, if that had been true.

"Our hands were shaking so much we couldn't dial our cell phones. So my daughter and I put our heads out of a window and screamed 'Help, help', as loudly as we could." This frightened the burglars, who ran up the road to a waiting getaway car. They got a screen from her computer and the DVD player, but not much else.

Hendriks, Baleta, and her daughter had just become part of the statistics that showed that violent crime in South Africa was running at a staggering 500 000, a year in which 20 000 were murders and another 54 000 involved rape.

Larry had cuts and bruises and refused to go to hospital. He was just treated by the paramedics who came with the police.

"I don't suppose they will ever catch them," Baleta said, in a forlorn sort of way.

The intruders had entered the house by smashing the wooden front door to pieces with their hammers. They could not have done it without making a deafening noise, but, as they had planned, it was muffled by the storm.

By the time I arrived, the house was being turned into a fortress like thousands of other South African homes. Steel security gates had already been bolted on the walls outside the front door and at the bottom of the stairs. Crime was now so rampant that even making your home as impenetrable as Fort Knox did not guarantee your safety.

Baleta was managing the stores section of an electrical wholesaler in 2000, when she developed a "terribly sore back." She believed this was caused by helping to lift heavy boxes from time to time as part of her job.

Through her firm she was covered by a good medical aid scheme, so she went to the nearby Mulbarton private hospital. After she had an MRI scan there, orthopedic surgeon Dr. Corrie Burger diagnosed a slipped disc. Traction she had did not help. As the pain just got worse, Dr. Burger decided to refer her to a spinal specialist. Fate then made its first devilish move. "The first doctor he had in mind had contracted out of medical aid so he said I must see Dr. Lieberthal, because he charged medical aid rates," said Baleta.

Noticeably thin, her pale face framed by long curly brown hair was etched by years of physical and mental suffering. I was soon to find out the reason why she could not sit for long.

She got a glimpse into the character of the doctor she had put her trust in before he had even examined her. "The first time I saw Dr. Lieberthal, he was standing in his reception area talking to his receptionist about his new Porsche that had just been delivered."

In his rooms, she sat down opposite him and put the envelope containing her MRI x-rays on the desk in front of her. She had not looked inside the envelope, as she preferred to leave that to the doctors. He gave her a quick examination in a cubicle before she returned to his desk.

Fate was hovering above her again, ominously ready to play another dirty trick on her. "When I came out, he had my MRI"s laid out on his desk. With his pen, he had circled the place on one of them that he said showed where I had a slipped disc in my lower back. He said I needed a fusion. 'It's urgent,' he said. 'If you don't have it done, you're going to be crippled'."

Her expression showed just how stressful it was to recall these events that had happened seven years earlier. "I immediately panicked. I asked if there was a possibility of there being any complications afterwards and he guaranteed that my recovery would be one hundred percent. At no stage did he tell me that the fusion might fail or that I could have even worse back pain after the operation."

This was Baleta's first back operation, so she was terribly nervous when Hendriks took her to the Rosebank Clinic one afternoon in July 2000. "I nearly cancelled," she said, recalling the moment with some trepidation. "As Larry was dropping me off, I told him, 'I can't stay here. I don't want to stay here. I don't want this operation.' I was in a real state. He said, 'Just go in and speak to the doctor when he comes to see you in the morning and take it from there.'" She soon found out that was easier said than done.

There were things she wanted to ask Dr. Lieberthal before he operated, to try and put her mind at rest. "'Where's the doctor? Where's the doctor?' I kept asking the nurses. 'No, you'll see him now, he's coming now.' When the anesthetist came to see me just before the operation, I said, 'Please I want to speak to the doctor.' He assured me he would call him. Eventually, as I was being wheeled to theatre, I again asked to speak to the doctor. 'No, you'll see him now.' Then the injection took over and before I knew it, I was gone. I think, I saw him only once after the operation."

According to Lieberthal's invoice, she had fusions at several levels of her spine, even though she was told that she only had one slipped disc. This involved having screws and other hardware inserted to hold everything together while the bone graft knitted. The bone for the graft was taken from her thigh.

Five days later, she was allowed home, but to her consternation the improvement that Lieberthal had promised never materialized. So she was readmitted to hospital for pain control. "Dr. Lieberthal had gone somewhere, so he never saw me. He just booked me in and said they must put me on a drip."

To make matters worse for Baleta, she had to contend with a most upsetting situation right there in the ward, where she was trying to recover. "There was this black lady who was from Swaziland, I think. She was crying her eyes out. She was fighting with the nurses. Loudly, so we could all hear, she yelled, 'He's crippled my daughter. She's only nine. Can he not come and see me?'" Baleta added.

She was almost certainly talking about Mrs. Mashanini. In the statement from Sister Maria Rapoo that Lieberthal submitted to the Nursing Council, she was supposed to have claimed that Sister Theunissen told a student nurse to tell Samantha Mashanini's mother that Lieberthal had "messed her daughter up."

The child was in Baleta's ward, although she did not see much of her because the curtains around her bed were usually closed. She got talking to the girl's mother who told her, "This doctor just doesn't want to come and see us. She walked in here and she's now a cripple." Jacqui gathered the little girl was paralyzed from the waist down.

What she heard next showed that Lieberthal's callousness had evidently rubbed off on some of the staff who worked with him. "A nurse said to this woman, 'Well, just go back home'. This made her even more agitated, and she screamed back at the nurses, 'She says that I must take my daughter back crippled.' I then told her I had been asking for Dr. Lieberthal day in and day out, and every time they would send somebody else."

That was the kind of treatment you might easily get in a government hospital, not usually in a private one, so I asked, "We are talking about in the Rosebank Clinic, are we?"

"Yes," she replied. "I said to the nurses, 'Why can't I see Dr. Lieberthal? I need to speak to him. He's the one who did my operation.' 'No, he's very busy.'"

"So you never saw him then or when you went back in for pain control?" I inquired.

"No. It was the same story as just before my operation."

The pain control was only temporary. "Three months after the operation I was still in absolutely agony. It was worse than before I first went into hospital."

She phoned Lieberthal. As usual, he was not to blame. "He told me I must have fallen and damaged the screws. I argued with him. 'I haven't fallen,' I said. 'Just come in,' he replied, 'and have some x-rays done, and I'll book you for another operation to put in bigger screws.'"

Our far-sighted specialist had already decided she needed another operation just by cross-examining her on the phone. After that, she saw him again and had further x-rays done. "He wanted to operate again because he said some of the screws he had put in had worked loose. I would have to wait two weeks as he would be in Australia." He booked her to have the second operation at the end of October 2000.

Her partner's friend was Dr. Matthew Leisher, a local GP. She was due to go back into the Rosebank Clinic on the Sunday. On the Friday, Leisher phoned to warn her against going back to Dr. Lieberthal. "He suggested I should get a second opinion from Dr. Percy Miller, a neurosurgeon at the Linksfield Park Clinic. So I cancelled my Rosebank admission, and I never heard from Dr. Lieberthal again."

Her story got a lot more hair-raising the more she went on. A few days later, Baleta was seeing Dr. Miller for another assessment. She handed him her envelope of MRI x-rays, which she got back from the Rosebank Clinic when she left hospital. He opened the envelope, and that's when Baleta, who was already run down because of all her harrowing experiences in the previous few months, got the biggest shock of all.

She could not believe it. How could Dr. Lieberthal have done such a thing? must have been going through her mind over and over again, like a stuck CD.

"'This isn't your MRI,' Dr. Miller told me. 'It is,' I said, 'it's got the circle which Lieberthal put on it with his pen to show me where he was going to operate.'

"Can you imagine how I felt when he said, 'But look at the name on the top? That's not yours.' My MRI's were there with somebody else's."

There were four MRIs in the envelope, two of which were hers and the other two had the name of a Mr. Economou on the top, and it was on one of the Economou ones that Lieberthal had drawn the circle. They had been taken by an entirely different radiology practice to the one where Baleta had gone.

"Dr. Lieberthal had done my operation based on Economou's MRIs and, after comparing these with my ones, Dr. Miller told me that I shouldn't have had a spinal fusion," she said. "All I needed was just three injections. This other guy should have got the operation I had."

Miller told her Lieberthal had put the screws in her nerves on the one side and, on the other side, a screw wasn't screwed into anything. It was just hanging there.

"Dr. Miller undertook to fix me up. He said the operation would take about an hour. But it took six and a half hours because it was only once he opened me up that he saw what a mess there was inside."

"Were you on a lot of medication after that?" I asked.

"Thank the Lord, I got over those pills. I just take over-the-counter pills now, nothing that requires a prescription. I was being messed up psychologically with pain pills, anti-depressants, steroids, and anti-inflammatories. I think I used to take about eighteen pills at a time."

Patting her Chihuahua, sitting on a cushion on the desk in front of her, she said, "It's this dog Tinkles that helped me get off all the medication."

"How long have you had her?"

"About three years, hey, Tinks?" She was a throwaway dog. A couple who had been staying in the backyard of one of their friends broke up and left her behind. "Our friends had their own dog, so they didn't want another one and when we went to visit, she just attached herself to me."

Baleta had been unaware that, if she wanted to sue Lieberthal for negligence, she had three years in which to do it. The time was ticking away, and it looked as though she would lose out. Then her mother came to the rescue.

"My mother, who lives in Stutterheim in the Eastern Cape, has a lawyer friend. One day she phoned me in a panic. 'Quick, quick,' she said. 'You've only got a short time left. You must go and see Stephen Flowers.' So I did, and he said I stood a very good chance because I've got good evidence."

Flowers took on her case on a no-win, no-fee basis, because Baleta certainly did not have the money to mount any kind of legal action.

Lieberthal settled out of court. No doubt all the media hype had helped to prepare the way for people like Baleta to get compensated without a long, drawn out case. She was left with R1.2-million after deducting the attorney's fee and other expenses.

She lost the job she had held for fourteen years because of her back problems.

"If you think loyalty gets you somewhere, it doesn't," was her sad comment. "If you want loyalty, get a dog," she added, giving Tinks a pat. She bought a cutter and started her own vinyl sign business working from home.

Anticipating that her prospects were grim, I asked, "How are you now?"

"I battle with pain permanently. I can't sit or stand for long. I'm just messed up and they say I've got to go for further back operations when the part they've screwed wears out. Then they've got to do it again, and so on and so on."

At the time Dr. Miller operated on her, he had been one of four specialists in private practice, who received kickbacks for referring patients to radiologists Illes and Partners between 1994 and 1999. A total of R2.65-million was paid to the referring doctors. In 2004, Miller and two of the others were found guilty by the HPC and he was fined R765 153. This was said to be equal to the kickback amounts he had received. It was hardly a punishment, as it meant he had the use of the money interest-free for up to five years.

Like Lieberthal, he was also required to work in the public service as part of the penalty, but, in his case, he only had to do it for one day a week for two years.

Miller claimed he had not knowingly done anything wrong. On his website, he maintained that "No patient or medical aid ever suffered from our actions, which ultimately came down to some sort of fee-splitting arrangement—the radiological bill was the same—only some of it went to us, whether legally or illegally, knowingly or unknowingly, is beside the point."

Neurologist Dr. Stanley Levy was the worst offender among the doctors. He was practicing in Australia by the time the matter was finalized, having been given a Certificate of Good Standing by the HPC, evidently as a reward for ratting on his colleagues. He admitted to receiving R882 690 from the radiologists, three of whom pleaded guilty to overbilling and creating perverse incentives. They were suspended from practicing for between 3 and 18 months and had to pay various fines.

No guilty finding was ever made against Levy, and nor did he have to repay the money he got, after he changed his original statement and gave evidence that there was no formal business venture between the doctors, and Illes and Partners, which might well have got them off the hook.

Chapter 21

Doctor Protection Council

Another particularly glaring example of how the Health Professions Council protected Lieberthal occurred more than two years before he was exposed for what he was by the media. The experience of Sheila Ball showed Lieberthal could well have continued messing up people's backs, while the compliant Medical Council went on throwing out complaint after complaint.

At 48, when she was working as a secretary, Sheila consulted her GP, Dr. Maureen Woolf in Blairgowrie, the middle-class suburb of Johannesburg where she was living. "I had a neck problem and I couldn't turn my head," she told me. "I had a few twinges in my back, but that wasn't bad, by any means."

She was referred to Lieberthal. "Maureen, who had been my GP for a long time, said he's an excellent back surgeon and when you see "Specialist in spinal disorders", you're impressed. He had that on his door. Three times he said to me, 'Imagine life without pain'. I thought, that sounds very attractive."

Lieberthal operated on her neck and lower back under one anesthetic. He took bone from her hip for the bone graft and did a fusion at four levels in her neck and three in her lumbar region. After five days, she was discharged from hospital in a wheelchair and told to come back for a check-up in six weeks' time.

She was not impressed by Lieberthal's habit of calling his patients by their first name. "He's probably one of the few doctors who have ever called me by my first name. You know, you are usually Mrs. But in turn, he liked to be called Wynne. So we were really pally-pally. He puts you at ease. The first meeting I had with him was long; he gave me all his time. That was the only time he was nice, if you like."

He left things lying on his desk which she couldn't help looking at while he was busy on the phone and they were all about "money and property" and that "sort of thing." "He had no interest in you at all after the first meeting."

She complained that on the morning of the operation she never saw him. "He didn't sort of greet you as you go in. That human touch did not exist. To me, it was very scary because my only other recollection of operations was successful ones, when I was in the most capable hands. He had no compassion. I had two blackouts after I returned home and he just wrote out another prescription. It just goes to show how wrong you can be.

"All his patients in the ward were there for redoes. There were six of them altogether. And he would talk to me about some of them behind their backs, which I thought was incredibly unprofessional. 'Oh, no, she's just a pain. She's just neurotic and she's this….' What made it worse was that he named the women he was talking about."

After the operation she was in terrible pain, and her father, Peter, who had come up from George to help this mother of two, tried to get hold of Lieberthal. "It was Jewish holidays, and he had gone over to the U.K.," she said. "Dr. Szabo was his second in command. I had never seen him before. He prescribed the strongest pain killers, little red things which didn't touch sides. You can tell a Lieberthal patient, I found out subsequently, by the drugs you are just doled out with at the end."

She was unable to sit, walk or even get out of bed, the pain was so intense. From a healthy 61 kg woman, she went down to 48 kilos in two weeks. "I was just skin on a frame. It was very scary. About three weeks after I had left the Rosebank Clinic, I was admitted to Olivedale Clinic still in a wheelchair.

"My leg was huge, and I was in so much pain with my back that I couldn't really care about the leg; but my dad was worried. He knew what it was, and he contacted Maureen Woolf." Her GP managed to get her an emergency appointment with Paul Cooke, a cardiovascular specialist.

"His face just dropped when he looked at my leg and he said, 'Admit her straight away.' Of course, that sent my poor heart into a frenzy. I thought, 'Oh no, now what's wrong?'" Ball had a deep vein thrombosis in her leg, which was successfully treated with Warfarin to thin her blood.

Three months later, she was readmitted to the Rosebank Clinic for pain control. "They gave me a shot of Pethidine," she said with a dreamy look. "It was the most amazing feeling. This was the first time since the operation that I was free of pain. On the second day, Lieberthal breezed in and out and said I was doing very, very well, as he always did. At one stage he said I must not have any physio. Then he changed his mind. But the physiotherapist could never get hold of him to find out what she had to do. So I never had it."

Her husband, a structural engineer, who had worked for Goldfields, a leading global gold mining house, never met Lieberthal, which was probably just as well. "He said, 'If I do, I'll kill him'," she told me. "Oh no, it was a very bad experience."

A year after Lieberthal operated on her she went back to him, after she had consulted four other specialists, Dr. Snyckers, Dr. Edeling, Dr. Craig, and Dr. Zwonnikoff.

"Why was that?" I asked.

"I wanted him to confirm to me my worst fears, and that was that both parts of my spine needed to be done again because he hadn't done it properly the first time." She had no intention of letting him do another operation. Her dad was with her as a witness when Lieberthal admitted that both needed to be redone. The x-rays they discussed showed how a screw that was supposed to have gone into the pedicle bone had missed it completely. "He just glossed over this when I asked him about it," she commented.

Having examined Mrs. Ball's x-rays, Dr. Craig concluded that the largest disc protrusion at the C3-C4 level was left untreated and there were screws that had been misplaced. He wrote that the "wide total laminectomy" at three levels of her lower back was "surprising since the patient showed no evidence of stenosis or other nerve root compression pathology."

She showed me her x-rays taken after the operation. There were rods in her back with a crossbeam, making them look like rugby goal posts; only the cross beam had come adrift on the one side. It made me shiver to think that she had been going around with this loose metal rod in her back for nine years because that was how long ago the operation had taken place when I saw her. She had a metal plate in her neck which had not been put in straight.

Mrs. Ball was particularly shocked by what Dr. Zwonnikoff had to say about the operation that cost R80 000. "He said the only time he had ever come across a case similar to mine, where two spine operations were done at the same time, with not such an extensive fusion as mine, the guy died."

On her readmission to Rosebank Clinic, there was a woman in her thirties in the bed next to her and Lieberthal had done nine operations on her. "She loved being sick," Sheila told me. "She really wanted the attention. Her body was in a ghastly state, she was so thin. It scared me that he had done so many operations on her. It was like 'One flew over the cuckoo's nest'. Do you remember that film? I made a conscious effort then; you know you have to take control. I wasn't sure how I was going to do it. Anyway, I slowly but surely got back into a healthy body again and put on some weight. I've worked on getting fit. My best friends are exercise and my yoga." She had, however, been unable to return to work as a typist because sitting for long periods put too much strain on her back.

Since her operations, Ball had seen Woolf, her GP, in passing. "I think she feels bad, but I don't blame her at all. She had a patient who thought Lieberthal was wonderful and then the husband or partner went to him, as well. So that's why she recommended him to me, but she vowed she would not send anybody else to him after what happened to me."

Woolf suggested she should sue Lieberthal, but she did not want to be involved in a long court case. She felt money would not bring back what Lieberthal had taken away. "I just wanted to stop him doing to others what he had done to me."

Her campaign to get the Health Professions Council to take action against Lieberthal began in September 1999 and ended in August 2001. She finally gave up when it was clear that Lieberthal could do no wrong in the Council's eyes.

All she got was disgusting service and a depressing picture of Lieberthal being given preferential treatment at every turn.

The surgeon was allowed to submit his reply to her complaint five months after the deadline the Council had set. It was not even persuaded that Lieberthal had done anything wrong by a letter she sent in January 2000 from Dr. Michael Kramer, the Ombudsman for the Gauteng Branch of the South African Medical Association. In it he stated, "That this type of major spinal surgery, namely anterior cervical fusion plus lumbar decompression and fusion under the same anesthetic does not constitute acceptable orthopedic practice."

Lieberthal's favorable treatment was such that, after the Committee of Preliminary inquiry considered the five-page attorney's letter submitted in his Defense, it decided to "consult" him personally at its next hearing. Ball was told that she would be "notified when and at which venue the next meeting would be held." This implied she could attend, but complainants are never given this opportunity in the early stages of one of these inquiries.

Everything is loaded in favor of doctors. Why embarrass them unnecessarily by having their accusers there? It was like having a court case without the victim being present. The Council had apparently not heard of the maxim: Justice should be seen to be done.

This was a perfect example of the Council's one-sided justice. Lieberthal was given two bites of the cherry, with the second one being an interview without Ball being there to refute or agree with what he said.

Lieberthal was completely innocent of any wrongdoing, his attorney maintained in the letter he sent to the Medical Council. "Dr. Lieberthal takes exception to Mrs. Ball's allegation that she had sought several professional opinions and the general consensus was that the procedure performed on the cervical spine had been unsuccessful, and the operation on the lumbar spine was totally unnecessary. He is confident that both procedures were well indicated and that the procedures were performed with the required level of expertise. Dr. Lieberthal treated Mrs. Ball throughout like a diligent and conscientious orthopedic surgeon."

Were Lieberthal's peers, who decided that all these things were perfectly acceptable, setting a new standard in orthopedic practice?

Was doing two extensive procedures under one anesthetic all right in their eyes? Was it fine to put a screw in that missed the bone completely? Was it good practice to do a wide laminectomy when there was no evidence to warrant it?

"What did you think about the way the Medical Council dealt with your complaint?" I asked Mrs. Ball.

"It was disgusting. He's a very talented man with words. I would be no match for him. Without 702 and The Star he could probably still be working undercover."

Mrs. Ball's initial symptoms and the operation Lieberthal did on her were virtually replicas of what happened to Piet Strauss: Only the treatment she got from the Medical Council was even shabbier. The Council was evidently in its Lieberthal can do no wrong phase when the complaints from both of them arrived in Pretoria. That was when the Council was still comfortably out of the searchlight of publicity that suddenly illuminated its terrifying shortcomings not long afterwards.

How was the treatment meted out to Lieberthal in these two cases different from a malpractice point of view, compared with the seven for which he was struck off the register? In both cases, the Council found Lieberthal had done nothing wrong, yet Strauss was awarded substantial damages when he sued Lieberthal.

Talk about double standards or perhaps no standards at all.

Bekink was one of the people, and no doubt there were others, who missed the bus completely when it came to suing Lieberthal for a substantial amount of money. On the face of it, she had an excellent case, but she lost out through ignorance of the law. The slothful workings of the Medical Council didn't help her, either.

In his court case to stop Radio 702 from defaming him, she was the woman Lieberthal stated under oath that he did not recognize when she phoned into the station. This was a lie, as my conversation with her showed.

As Strauss said, she was in "dire straits" and this certainly was the case when I saw her. She got divorced 26 years earlier because she was what she described as a "battered wife." She had two grown-up children, Debbie and Warren, both of whom were married and living in KwaZulu-Natal. Neither of them was in a position to give her much financial help or take her in. She was clearly very lonely. "I don't get many visitors," she told me, shooing her three dogs out of the way into the back room. Bow, Jodi, and Terry, a fox terrier, a Labrador, and one of an indeterminate breed, were her only companions.

Bekink had worked for the South African Broadcasting Corporation in Johannesburg as a receptionist for 13 years when her chair collapsed and the back of it hit her spine as she fell. After that, she had three back operations by different surgeons. When she was no better, a colleague at work suggested she see Lieberthal, who the woman described as "fantastic."

She went to see him in July 1997 just after she was retrenched by the SABC.

"Why were you retrenched," I inquired.

"First of all, if you were 50 years and older, they retrenched you if you were white. If you had 10 years or more service, they retrenched you. They were getting rid of all the old girls, old people basically. What I paid in for my pension, I got out. I had to live off that for a while and when I was 53, I got a government disability pension."

At her first consultation with Lieberthal, he said, "Oh, good heavens, he's got screws in there that are so big. You don't need screws that size." He was talking about the ones inserted by one or more of her three previous surgeons.

"I don't know if you've seen his card," she said, moving to a new position on the couch. "When he tells you that, you think he knows what he's talking about. So he said these had to come out. He was the owner of a screw company and he wanted to use his screws in my back. That's how it all came about."

The 24 operations Lieberthal did on her back between 1997 and 2000 cost over a million rand. All of them were paid for by Workman's Compensation, a division of the Department of Labour that assists people injured in the workplace. They were to put in or take out screws and other hardware or to clean out the wound that had become infected. In total, she was in hospital for 207 days. She had a plastic bag containing 38 screws, some as long as seven centimeters, and 17 assorted bars and rods that had been removed.

"I can't believe that he did so many operations on you," I said.

"Yes, nobody can."

"What I can't understand is why you kept going back to him?"

"After the first couple, there was pus coming out of my back, and nobody else wanted to clean up another doctor's mess. He never fixed me up. When I would go back, he would open me up and take out all the rods and crews because of the infection. I was doubling over because my back got so weak. When the rods were in to hold me up, it was brilliant.

"He seemed to have a reasonable bedside manner, put it that way, to begin with. But as things went on, he was pathetic. There were many times in hospital when the nurses tried to get hold of him when things weren't right and the pus was pouring out of the wound in my back. I'm not the only one; there's been many, many complaints. When you tried to get hold of him, particularly on a weekend, he was either away or he wasn't available. Somehow or other, you couldn't pin him down, that's for sure. Sometimes he would leave messages for the nurses to do this or that. Then he would see you on Monday morning and you had to be grateful to see him sort of thing."

Getting off the couch, she crawled to the bedroom to fetch something, leaving her elbow crutches behind her. When she returned, she said, "I'm going to sit on the floor, if you don't mind."

"Have you got any rods in your back now?" I asked, because she looked like a hunchback, extremely bent over.

"Nothing, that's why I'm like this," she added tearfully. "I've got nothing to hold me up."

"Why did he take them all out then?"

"No, Dr. Zwonnikoff took them out because of the infection in the wound. I saw him because Workman's Compensation refused to allow me to go back to Dr. Lieberthal. They weren't prepared to pay for more ops by him."

That was her 28th back operation.

Nonplussed, I said, "What I can't understand is if the rods were holding you up, why did Zwonnikoff take them out?"

"Because my whole body was being poisoned by the infection. Home nurses were coming here twice a day to change my bedding because the bath towel and the pillow I had under me was wet with pus that was coming out of my back. It was bad, very bad."

Reporting on the operation he did in January 2001, Zwonnikoff wrote: "There were extensive areas of sepses in the deep muscle layer and the entire hardware system, consisting of 10 screws and two longitudinal rods, were removed. It was clear that sepses were coming from around the screws themselves."

I gathered that on a much larger scale, it was like having a thorn in your foot that was causing an infection. The problem would not clear up until the thorn was removed.

"How many times did you get an infection after Lieberthal's operations?"

"Oh gosh, I'm not sure, at least five times."

"Did Zwonnikoff tell you the only way of curing it was to remove the rods?"

"Yes, and since then, I'm clean. I've had several tests done at the Johannesburg General Hospital and the infection has gone."

When I saw her she was pinning her hopes of having her back straightened on another operation done by Zwonnikoff to insert screws and other hardware once again. It was as though Lieberthal had put her in some kind of medieval torture rack from which there was no easy escape.

"That's the next best bet because, without assistance, I can't stand up," she added.

Her major stumbling block was that Workman's Compensation had turned off the money supply. The regulations stipulated that the Commissioner "shall for a period not exceeding two years from the date of the accident be liable for the reasonable medical expenses incurred by the workman." After that, it was left to the Commissioner's discretion to pay for further treatment, which would reduce the disablement.

Bekink did not take "No" for an answer. She asked for help from the National Ombudsman, Advocate Lawrence Mushwana. Through his office, an appeal was lodged against the Commissioner's decision to close her file; and Lieberthal was subpoenaed to appear at the inquiry.

A review of her case in July 2006 by an anonymous "legal representative" stated, "Unfortunately, at the time of the hearing, several complaints had been laid against Dr. Lieberthal with the Health Professions Council. It is understandable that the panel could not place particular weight on his testimony. I am not a medical practitioner and do not purport to have an intimate knowledge of the patient's condition, but it would appear from all the documents I studied at the Compensation Commissioner, that many of the operations were totally unnecessary. Dr. Lieberthal, however, was of the opinion that a further operation would be beneficial to the patient and would improve her condition. He was very sure of this.

"Dr. Zwonnikoff appeared uncertain of the chances of success and improvement of the patient after the requested operation. Although his testimony was that he would assist, it appeared from cross-examination that he did not really want to perform the operation personally. This is unfortunate, as the medical practitioners testifying on behalf of the Commissioner were adamant that they did not rate the chances of success very highly.

"Dr. Charles Lautenbach, an orthopedic surgeon, who gave evidence on behalf of the Commissioner, believed that Bekink needed 'psychiatric help' and he was attempting to wean her off her 'very heavy consumption of non-steroid and anti-inflator drugs'. He certainly didn't help her case when he said, 'The bending of the back is not a result of the un-united fracture of the back but appears to be mainly occurring at the bending of the hips'."

He was in favor of treating her conservatively for depression and, more importantly, to help her to "accept her pain."

The legal report emphasized that the Commissioner had to be satisfied that the patient's disability would be reduced before agreeing to pay for any more treatment. "From the testimony at the hearing," it went on, "for and against re-opening the file, the panel could not have come to any other decision than to uphold the refusal of the Commissioner."

Bekink was left with a jelly-like back, with very little prospect of being able to get anybody to pay to have it strengthened with more metal rods, and the like.

In a letter he wrote to the Professor of Orthopedic Surgery at the Johannesburg General Hospital, Zwonnikoff appealed to him to "help this unfortunate lady" by taking over the management of her case.

Criticizing Workman's Compensation he wrote, "She was originally a WC case; however, with the usual lack of co-operation on the part of the Workman's Compensation Commissioner, Mrs. Bekink has reached an impasse in terms of funding her future investigations or treatment."

Bekink now had nobody to pay for the operation she so fervently believed would straighten her back. When I saw her for the last time, the infection had returned. Ever the optimist, she was still hoping that Workman's Compensation would pay for another operation. She had been assessed as only 50 percent disabled. This meant she was trying to survive on a monthly pension of R1 700. She had been dipping into the access bond of R100 000 she had on her little, dilapidated house which, at best, was worth around R400 000 and had come to the end of this.

While Bekink was concentrating on trying to get her Workman's Compensation case reopened, vital time was slipping by. She, like Baleta, was unaware that if she wanted to bring an action for damages against Lieberthal summons had to be issued against him within three years from the time when she first became aware of the problem.

That was the law in South Africa and, if nothing was done in the three-year period, the case became proscribed. Unfortunately, she did not know anybody who would have tipped her off about this.

The Radio 702"s expose` of Lieberthal's screw-ups, which she heard in 2002, prompted her to send a letter to the Health Profession Council saying that she believed that, had he done the first operation properly, the rest would not have been necessary. She got an acknowledgement of her complaint in October 2002. Nine months later, the Council sent her another letter, saying that it had been decided to hold an inquiry into Lieberthal's conduct.

In its inefficient way, the Council never bothered to send her the result. Five years after she made her complaint, I contacted the HPC with a letter of authority from her. I asked what had been decided about her complaint. The reply I received from Tendai Dhliwayo, the Council's Communications Officer, was, "The complaint was finalized in July 2004. The doctor was found guilty and sentenced to an effective erasure from the register."

No wonder newspapers get things wrong at times, when you have public relations officers feeding them with this kind of information. This result did not refer to Bekink's case at all. It was what happened after Lieberthal's disciplinary hearing involving the seven totally unrelated charges.

When I queried this, he told me that there had been about 20 complaints Lieberthal had to face, but it had been decided to try him on the seven strongest ones initially. If these had not resulted in him being struck off, they would have charged him with the remainder, one of which had been Bekink's. Not keeping her in the picture was inexcusable.

Had the Council got a move on with Bekink's case and given her a guilty finding against Lieberthal reasonably soon after she complained, it might have prompted her to go to an attorney in time. Consequently, it was only after she heard about how other people had successfully sued Lieberthal that she realized she also had a good case. For her, it was too late. All the lawyers she consulted told her that, as the three-year period had elapsed, her claim had proscribed.

"I believed I could have got at least two million," she told me tearfully.

Ignorance of the law is no excuse, the saying goes, but should this apply in cases like Bekink's? How was she and possibly others like her supposed to know about the three-year proscription period, when she had no legal knowledge and had never been involved in anything like this before?

Chapter 22

Reformed Character

In October 2006, just over two years after he had been struck off, Lieberthal decided it was time to become a respected surgeon again, so he applied to the Health Professions Council to be reinstated. He was on his knees, presenting himself as a man very different from the stroppy, defiant character that he was at his disciplinary inquiry. His application letter was addressed to Advocate Mkhize, the man he had bitterly attacked at his hearing.

He began by giving what he called an "overview" of his career. He listed all the prizes he had won as a registrar and mentioned that in 2002 he had been "nominated for the Phyllis Knocker/Bradlow Award for achievements in surgery."

The monetary award of R45 000 is made to Fellows of the College of Medicine of South Africa who not only achieved exceptional results in the final Fellowship examination, but whose professional careers have shown "evidence of valuable contributions to basic or clinical research, participation in community health projects, or the advancement of the humanitarian aspects of medical or dental practice."

Lieberthal was the antithesis of what the award stood for, yet, according to Mrs. Ann Vorster, the Academic Registrar of the CMSA, he was not nominated, but invited to submit his research protocol because he had done sufficiently well in the examinations. He did not win the award.

All Fellows who have passed their final written and oral examinations are asked to submit their research protocol for evaluation by a panel of the Examinations and Credentials Committee. In 2002 this, no doubt, took place shortly before Lieberthal's image was horribly disfigured by the media later that year. Even then, I would have thought that, by the time he was asked to submit his name, those heavyweight dignitaries on the Committee would have had their ears close enough to the ground to have heard the scandalous talk about Lieberthal. At that stage, it must have spread through medical circles like measles at a kindergarten.

In his letter, Lieberthal embellished his story about winning the "Surgeon

General's Medal for meritorious service." He was the "first national serviceman to be awarded this medal." This was another one of his lies because there was never any such medal when he claimed to have won it. In fact, in his statement giving the causes of his insolvency in 1991, he wrote, in his own handwriting, that he had received the "Surgeon General's award for meritorious service while on active duty." On this occasion, he did not refer to it as a medal so it appeared to be a reference to the Certificate he received, a copy of which he included in documents he submitted to court when he sued Netcare.

Major John Keene, the chief curator of the South African National Military History Museum in Johannesburg and a member of the SADF Medal Advisory panel, substantiated what the 32 Battalion veterans had told me when he said, "I can say without hesitation there was no official medal by that name awarded. There was the South African Medical Services Cross, but that only came into being in 1994."

Lieberthal gave details of his various achievements early in his career. Following his National Service, he did further training as a senior medical officer in the Department of Surgery at Wits University, where he rotated through the following disciplines: trauma; pediatric surgery; cardiothoracic surgery, and urology. This was before he started his own GP practice in 1985.

In 1996, he graduated as "the best orthopaedic registrar in the country and was awarded the Jock Edelstein Medal of the College of Orthopaedic Surgeons for this."

Then he was put in charge of spinal surgery at the Johannesburg Hospital. He also performed and taught surgery at other teaching hospitals affiliated to the University of the Witwatersrand. At the same time, he was involved in the training of undergraduate medical students (lectures and clinical work), and postgraduate practical and theoretic training of orthopedic registrars and neurosurgeons. "It was generally reported back to the then academic head Prof. Erken, by registrars-in-training, that I was one of the best post-graduate teachers," he boasted.

The enigma that was Lieberthal told Mkhize his charitable work for the community involved conducting a spinal deformities outpatient clinic once a week at the Johannesburg Hospital; teaching the registrars weekly; and operating at one of the teaching hospitals at least once a week on a voluntary basis. "Until 2001, I received no salary from the state institutions," he declared. "Thereafter, I was paid on a sessional basis. I was frequently invited by other orthopedic surgeons in private practice to either assist them, or do their spinal surgery cases with and for them."

He had to make some reference to Sean Cooper, although he probably would have preferred not to mention him at all. A "tiny fragment of the tip of the scalpel blade" had broken off in a disc space, and both Cooper and his mother were fully informed about it immediately post-operatively. "I explained to them that the fragment posed no threat and I would monitor it on serial radiographs. Mr. Cooper even referred his brother to me for treatment." He stressed that Cooper's case was never one of the cases that were presented at his disciplinary hearing, as if that was a feather in his cap.

The Medical Defense Union had advised him to get Cooper to retract what he had said to the media in the presence of a witness. "I duly did this with Mr. Peter Cotterell, the then manager of the Rosebank Clinic. Mr. Cooper admitted to us that he had over-reacted and promised to withdraw the statement. However, he never did this."

I was not able to verify this with Cooper because he had already died when I began my inquiries for this book. I had to rely on his widow Tanya, as his mother and brother Justin were not prepared to co-operate.

"As far as I can remember, Sean was never, ever going to withdraw his statement," she said. "Lieberthal came into his ward at the hospital and begged him to withdraw it, but he didn't, as far as I know. The hospital then moved Sean into a private ward at their expense to basically keep him away from Lieberthal. They removed his name from the board outside. It was like he wasn't even a patient there."

Lieberthal didn't operate on Justin; she said he merely did an epidural which involved an injection into his spine. He was only in hospital for a day at the same time as Sean, and it was after Justin had been discharged that the news broke about the scalpel.

"It wasn't that it was after his operation that Sean recommended him, because there was no way in hell that anyone would recommend that doctor," she stressed.

I showed Cotterell the portion of Lieberthal's letter that referred to him and asked, "Do you have any recollection of that?"

"You know that was what, four years ago? There were a lot of things said round about that time."

"But this was obviously something you were specifically asked to witness."

"Did I sign anything?"

"No, I don't think so."

"I can't even say I can deny it, because God alone knows what was going on at that time. But there was nothing reduced to writing. I certainly didn't sign anything. I know Wynne Lieberthal was trying to accommodate Mr. Cooper."

"When you say "accommodate him", what do you mean?"

"Because whatever was published in The Star was through Sean Cooper, a colleague or whatever it was. It was Netcare's policy at the time to keep stories out of the Press at any cost."

"I find it difficult to believe that he would have got Cooper to agree to retract everything," I said.

"Wynne Lieberthal was the most charming guy. He could well have done. There was an old lady who had about 12 operations done by Lieberthal and she still said he was the most fantastic surgeon. I remember the matron telling me the story not long after I got there. I think he's a psychopath, but it doesn't stop them being excellent in one field," he added.

Cotterell had retired when I saw him. This undoubtedly accounted for the way he talked so freely about his hospital experience.

I told Tanya what Cotterell had said, and she replied, "That guy, excuse my French, was shitting himself, because I can tell you now, the little tearoom in the hospital was privately owned. And every single morning, the minute the newspapers got delivered, the hospital went and bought every single one. *Ja*, because when we went to buy one we were told the manager had come in and bought all the newspapers. You couldn't buy a newspaper in that hospital for like two weeks. That guy used to visit Sean on a daily basis. I remember him sitting in the private ward that the hospital was paying for, watching a rugby match on a Saturday afternoon like really sucking up to Sean."

In his plea to the Council, Lieberthal conceded that his efforts to stop the publicity he got by taking various legal actions "only served to spur the press and radio talk shows to air the story more widely and this, in turn, led to extensive coverage and debate publicly. My legal advice was to pursue the matter, and in retrospect I see that this only further inflamed matters."

The media exposure and having his "privileges" withdrawn by Netcare and other hospitals meant he was "unable to practice anywhere, despite not as yet having been found guilty or even having formal charges laid against me by the HPCSA"

This contrasted with the sworn affidavit he made when he brought that High Court action against the HPCSA in 2004. In it he stated: "I am presently only able to work on an ad hoc basis as a consultant for various state hospitals." Elsewhere in the letter, he wrote: "From October 2002, until now it has been impossible to make a living."

That was another phony claim. What about the million or so he earned from the Liberian job? And, at the end of his own letter, he said he had been working in the printing industry from the time he was struck off, possibly with his brother Hugh who had a printing business.

Playing for sympathy, he came up with this gem: "It has only been due to support from family, friends and charitable institutions that my family and I have managed to survive. I have lost all my assets and currently live in a rented home."

He again trotted out how his wife and five children had "borne the brunt of my financial and social embarrassment."

"Three of my children were in high school at the time that I was under such tremendous media pressure and they suffered terribly from the unrelenting, vicious coverage."

In spite of everything that had happened to him, he maintained: "I still have many calls from colleagues and former patients seeking my opinion and advice on treatment and management of cases. Many of my colleagues have made it clear to me that, should I be reinstated, they would not hesitate to make use of my expertise again. I would gladly supply a list of these colleagues." There were so many that he could only muster two of them to give him references. Predictably, the Medical Council did not ask for the list.

Attached to his letter were these references. One was from his long time promoter, Professor Erken, who was once again clapping and cheering him on, for some inexplicable reason, when he must have realized at that stage that Lieberthal should no longer be in medicine. "I warmly and strongly support his application for reinstatement without reservation," he wrote.

The other one was from orthopedic surgeon Nick Saragas, who stated: "In view of his excellent orthopedic knowledge, expertise and experience, his contribution will be extremely beneficial to the orthopedic community."

Lieberthal's next improbable statement was: "I have contacted former patients who I may have offended and apologized to them for my hurtful behavior." Why was it that, having spoken to many of them, I could not find one to whom he had said sorry?

"I am 51 years old and I would desperately like to be able to practice again, especially in a country such as ours, which needs orthopedic expertise," his plea continued. "I'm truly sorry for any harm or hurt I may have caused to anyone. The whole incident was just so out of character for me. Looking back at the hearing it is clear to me that I was ill advised by my legal advisers in several respects."

He rambled on about how his tremendous legal costs had all but exhausted his savings and assets when he had been unemployed prior to the hearing in 2004.

Coming to the tragic case of his advocate, Lieberthal implied that Goldblum's illness had been the reason why he had been found guilty at his disciplinary hearing. "Mr. Goldblum has a chronic, terminal illness, and this prevented him from preparing and defending me in the best possible manner. It was a serious consideration that he would be well enough and mentally sharp enough to provide a well-presented case on my behalf."

Why did he employ him then? The only logical explanation was that Goldblum was working for nothing or, alternatively, Lieberthal wanted a sick advocate so he could draw out the hearing with as many postponements as possible or both. He claimed that, although Goldblum had declared that he was acting pro bono on his behalf, this was not true "as he was receiving remuneration from me." What was his motive for making Goldblum out to be a liar when there was ample evidence that this was Lieberthal's specialty?

Did the HPCSA notice these obvious reflections on Lieberthal honesty, which were so well documented, when it considered his application to be restored to the register? All the indications were that the Council's approach seemed to have been, We don't have to doubt the truth of what our fellow doctors tell us, even if they have been struck off. After all, we are dealing with colleagues, honorable, professional people.

Lieberthal was not even required to make his application for reinstatement in a sworn affidavit form, which indicated that the Council trusted him to do the right thing or that, in its bumbling, it had never occurred to it that this might be necessary.

In my 2007 interview, I said to Mkhize, "These written submissions are not done in affidavit form, are they?"

"Not necessarily."

"Well, Lieberthal's wasn't. Shouldn't that be a requirement, because otherwise they can lie their heads off and it has no legal standing?"

"Well, people can also lie in an affidavit," he countered.

"Yes, but it's a criminal offence, is it not?"

"*Ja*, well, it will be perjury," he conceded. "We take the view that if there is an element of dishonesty in the submission, if that comes to light, it would have very dire and major consequences for the applicant."

"Well, you might be interested to know that Lieberthal's submission letter contained numerous half-truths and outright lies."

Looking somewhat shaken, he asked, "In what way?"

I then gave him an idea of what I had discovered. Conveniently, he could not recollect the details of the case. "I realize that," I said, "but what I'm trying to get at is, if somebody like Lieberthal puts in a five-page submission to be reinstated, and he tells the Council these are the facts of what he is putting forward in mitigation, does anybody check these things?"

He defended his Council with this flimsy explanation. "Well, there's a limited review process of the submissions that are made, not necessarily a full-blown one, but, like, getting confirmation here and there."

Despite Lieberthal's claim that he had specialists queuing up to work with him if he was reinstated, he had been unable to find a single one who was prepared to act as his expert witness at his disciplinary hearing.

Lieberthal described his decision to storm out of the hearing, and take the Council on review in the High Court as "an error of judgment", because he should have had "faith in the judgement" of the Committee trying him. He "deeply regretted" rushing into a legal dispute with the HPCSA, as this caused direct conflict with Mkhize and other members of the Council. "In the past few years I have had ample time to reconsider the course of action I elected to take, and am bitterly disappointed in myself for my rash and uncharacteristic behavior. I have most certainly learnt from this experience."

He admitted he had failed to consider his patients" point of view and their right to complain with the necessary "sympathy and insight required." He also accepted that he made errors in judgment in his treatment decisions. "For this I am truly sorry and I regret any pain I may have caused to any patient."

In case the Council got the idea that he might need the same kind of drug rehabilitation treatment he had received all those years before, when he was a trainee surgeon, he gave this assurance: "At the time and in the aftermath, I consulted a psychologist. At no time was medication prescribed or ongoing therapy thought to be necessary."

With a view to returning to practice, he had discussed the possibility of this with a number of colleagues, including Prof Erken, Prof Govender, who was a member of the Committee at his hearing, Prof Lukhele, and Prof K. Boffard, a member of the Board of the HPSCA. "All have expressed their support for my reinstatement."

Kenneth Boffard, the Professor of Surgery at Wits University, told me he had no recollection of having had such a discussion with Lieberthal. He had worked with him in the 1980s, at the Johannesburg Hospital, when Lieberthal trained many of the paramedics in what was then the Transvaal province, "and. I must say, he was damned good," he said, giving the surgeon a rare pat on the back.

I also asked Govender if he had supported Lieberthal's reinstatement and he said, "Aah, no. Let me put it this way, he told me about his dire financial consequences as a result of being struck off and he asked for my advice. I said to him, 'Look. You write to the Council.' That was it."

"That's hardly expressing your support, I would think," I said.

He chuckled before saying, "*Ja*, well. You can interpret it the way you want to, but I said to him, this is the Council's jurisdiction and you need to write to them."

Lukhele confirmed that Lieberthal had contacted him. But he too had not given Lieberthal any undertaking.

Our repentant surgeon finished his letter to Mkhize by saying, "I would like to apologize to any members and representative of the HPCSA who I may have offended with my rash behavior." He expressed a desire to attend his reinstatement hearing without his legal representative.

The man who could so easily cast a spell on his patients had an equally mesmerizing effect on the Medical Council. He got his way. He was reinstated on 16 January 2007. When I heard about what happened a month later. I put various questions to Tendai Dhliwayo at the Council. I asked what the factors were that made the Council decided to reinstate him?

He issued a statement listing all the fairly obvious things that the Council takes into account. These included, but were not necessarily limited to: "remorse; acknowledgement and appreciation of limitations and wrong doing; time elapsed between erasure and application for restoration; personal circumstances around the individual; potential to relapse; safeguards in place once the practitioner is restored; fitness to practice, etc." The Council found Lieberthal to have been "extremely remorseful in his submissions, both orally and in writing." He also acknowledged his weaknesses in pre- and post-operative management of patients.

The Council was satisfied that he had, of his own accord, gone back to his peers, whom he had offended and verbally attacked, to offer his apology. It also took into account that Lieberthal had lost almost all his assets as a result of the publicity his case generated in the media, which made him close his practice around 2002. Since when was losing your assets, because of your own nauseating behavior, a mitigating factor?

The next sentence made me doubt whether the Council members who heard his reinstatement application knew anything at all about the evidence given at his disciplinary hearing. "The Council also considered the fact that Lieberthal's medical skills had not been an issue, but that it was primarily around pre- and post-operative management of the patients," the statement went on. This was totally untrue on a par with a lot of Lieberthal's fantasies. It showed once again how far the Council was prepared to go to exonerate a "colleague."

Lieberthal was given his surgeon's title back on conditions that were similar to the ones that were imposed on him 16 years earlier. They were: that he practices under supervision only in the public service; that he undergoes training, the duration and content of which was to be determined by the Wits Medical School of Orthopedics; that he is trained in interaction with patients, and that his supervisor in the public service submits quarterly reports on his performance for a period of a year, after which the Council would reassess the position.

The Council showed its favoritism when his apology for the Irish Army sojourn was considered sufficient to erase that dubious episode. It also turned its blind eye to the allegations contained in my questions regarding Lieberthal's criminal activities. Were patients right in not expecting much protection from this body that was supposed to uphold the principles of the Hippocratic Oath and keep doctors in line?

After The Star newspaper reported that the Johannesburg Hospital was investigating Lieberthal for overcharging for hardware he used in his operations that had been bought from his own firm, the HPC was said to be doing its own investigation. I had asked what the result was of this investigation.

Revealing its lack of investigative expertise, as well as its half-hearted approach to cases of this kind, it did "not obtain evidence to confirm or sustain" these.

I also wanted to know if the HPC had ever investigated allegations made in Noseweek magazine about Lieberthal and others being involved in dubious dread disease insurance claims.

It seemed that the HPC only moved at all after receiving a complaint. No complaint automatically signified everything was rosy, even if an expose` appeared in a publication.

As had happened before, the Council just swept criminal allegations that did not have a direct connection to a patient under the very large carpet that the HPC appeared to keep for this very purpose.

My last question was: "In view of Lieberthal's record and the number of people who were maimed for life or left with permanent pain due to Lieberthal's treatment, what kind of message does the Council think it is sending to the public by reinstating him after less than three years?"

The answer showed once again that patients were regarded as second-class citizens, well behind doctors. "The HPCSA is quite cognizant of the fact that a number of patients may have had unpleasant and even life-threatening experiences as a result of contact with Dr. Lieberthal." Agonizing trauma was reduced to "unpleasant" by a Council that professed to have patients' welfare at heart. And how do you have "life-threatening experiences" when the doctor's only fault, according to the Council, was a poor bedside manner?

The real reason for allowing Lieberthal back into theatre then became apparent: There was a "severe doctor shortage in the country." Coupled with that, the Council was "always guided by such factors as to whether there are necessary safeguards in place to ensure that similar incidents do not recur in the future." In this instance, the members felt that their "limited restoration of Dr. Lieberthal is a measure which we believe will go a long way in both remedying his shortcomings, as well as making his skills available under supervision." The fact that similar restrictions imposed all those years before had not remedied his shortcomings did not seem to concern the Council at all.

The Council was satisfied he had "served his punishment" and his personal financial crisis attested to the kind of punishment he had to endure. The Council contended that by the time he was struck off in 2004, he had already served a punishment from 2002 when he had to close down his practice due to the high media publicity of his case. To support this view, it pointed to the courts where the time an individual spends in detention awaiting trial is often taken into account when they are sentenced.

Smugly congratulating each other on the way they had handled Lieberthal's reinstatement, the Council members announced that they were happy "with the remorse we have seen and his appreciation of his shortcomings." That made them "comfortable that he may be restored to the register." Lieberthal was still not employed in January 2007, as far as the Council was aware, because he had to obtain a post in the public service and submit the name of his supervisor.

The Council's press release concluded with more wise words designed to show that it was there, to impartially look after the interests of both doctors and their patients. "The message that we are sending is that doctors are human too and that they, like any of us, do sometimes commit mistakes and that the public has to understand this fact. Secondly, if you make a mistake, you will be punished and you will suffer just like Dr. Lieberthal suffered and continues to suffer. Thirdly, if there is sufficient evidence of remorse and, after a period of time serving your punishment, you may be considered for reinstatement. Above all, we are serious about professional misconduct and we will stop at nothing to deal with it."

It could not have been very comforting to many of Lieberthal's patients to hear that the Health Profession Council's philosophy regarding doctors was that human beings should not be written-off for life, when that was exactly what had happened to them at the hands of their surgeon. "Striking a doctor off the roll sent a very strong message," the Council's members declared. They cushioned this opinion by adding, "On the other hand, people do learn from their mistakes."

The Council showed a complete lack of compassion for Lieberthal's patients when it did not commiserate in any way with those who had suffered terribly as a result of the reckless way he wielded his scalpel.

Shortly after Lieberthal was reinstated, Dr. Feinberg, his one-time partner in his Lyndhurst GP practice, told me, "He still doesn't accept that he's done anything wrong. He was around here the other day. I never saw him, but he spoke to my nursing sister, Michele. She worked for him before I was involved in this practice. He said to her, 'You know what, I've done nothing wrong. They've prejudiced me unfairly'. I mean, when he worked with us as a partner you could bring him documents that he signed himself and he would tell you, 'Someone's forged my signature'. He's not prepared to take any responsibility for things that he creates and does himself. You know, he's a sick man. The story hasn't finished. It's only just begun, unfortunately. I'm loathed to see what's going to happen down the line. Not now, because he's going to work under supervision again. But once that terminates, wherever he goes, I shudder to think what's going to happen again."

Katopodis at 702 said, "I must admit I was completely gob smacked to hear Lieberthal had been reinstated as a doctor. How deeply disturbing! What's wrong with the HPCSA? Surely they are supposed to have the best interests of the public at heart. Many will argue that he has a right to earn a living and that he's paid his dues. I personally would have preferred it if he'd gone into another field altogether. I really don't believe that the medical fraternity needs, or wants, the likes of him in its ranks."

"Satan looks after his own," commented Ester, Mariskca du Plessis' mother.

"This is ridiculous," Tanya Cooper said when she heard the news. "I'm sending a letter of protest to the Health Professions Council. In the three months my husband was in hospital, I never met Lieberthal once and I was there nearly all the time."

According to the HPCSA's Form 115, the Board hearing an application for reinstatement has to consider various criteria in terms of the Health Profession Act. The document pointed out that the Board has the discretion to decide whether or not an applicant is a fit and proper person to be readmitted. "But this discretion will only be exercised in favor of restoration if it is satisfied that the evidence of reformation is overwhelming and that the

Board will not make a mistake if it readmits the applicant." How could the Council members who reinstated Lieberthal possibly have complied with this, if the information given in his application letter was never checked?

"During consideration of his application," the form stipulates, "cognizance will be had of his conduct over a period in order to establish whether he has completely reformed." How could the Council have complied with this, in view of the fact that, for almost half the time that Lieberthal was suspended, he was working for the Irish Army, a job he got by deception?

The regulations made it clear that the onus was on the applicant to prove that he had fully and permanently reformed. But how could a letter, without any evidence to support its contents, possibly be described as "proof?"

When I put it to Mkhize that the Council did not comply with the conditions laid down in the form he said, "There was compliance otherwise he would not have been reinstated."

Now that he had got his doctor's license back, would the Council's pet surgeon be able to find a hospital prepared to ignore his well-documented, monstrous record?

Chapter 23

Missing Surgeon

Seven months after Lieberthal was reinstated, I spoke to Professor Thanyani Mariba, the Chairman of the Medical and Dental Professions Board. This was the body that directly controlled doctors. It was represented on the Health Professions Council, which consisted of eleven boards for various branches of the medical profession. Mariba, a cardiologist, was Dean of the Faculty of Health Sciences at the University of Pretoria.

"At our meeting following his reinstatement," he said, "Dr. Lieberthal told us he went to Wits, and they wanted to employ him, but there was no post available."

What happened in fact was that there were three teaching hospitals, Johannesburg, Helen Joseph, and Baragwaneth, utilized by the Wits Medical School as part of its teaching circuit, where Lieberthal could have been employed. The only position available, which was suitable for him, was at Baragwaneth.

Professor George told me about a discussion that took place at one of their regular staff meetings. By this time, Professor Lukhele had succeeded him as head of the Orthopaedic section of the Wits Medical School. George was one of the few doctors I came across who was prepared to speak candidly about what went on in the inner sanctums of his profession. When I spoke to him, he had retired to Knysna on the Cape coast.

"Professor Lukhele read us a letter from the Medical Council," he said. "The Council had asked him to facilitate that Wynne Lieberthal will be installed as a doctor in an academic hospital under supervision. It was nothing against his surgical technique, the way he operated. The thing proved to him was that he was neglecting his patients."

"Well, that's rubbish," I retorted.

"*Ja*, I know. Professor Lukhele was very sympathetic, and he wanted him, really. As far as I know, he was appointed a principle medical officer at Baragwaneth Hospital. But I know from my senior colleagues they didn't want him there. You see, they were smelling that it's going to be a trouble. We were discussing it's going to be difficult because Dr. Lieberthal is too bright." He laughed. "He can cheat the system, that's the human dimension." Professor George did not feel inclined to join the objectors because he had been so close to retirement.

Mariba told me that after he realized Lieberthal could not get a job through the Wits Medical School, he took matters into his own hands. "I said look, I'll try and see if I can't help him. I'll phone around and see if there's somebody prepared to give him a job, even if it's a medical officer's job, so that the man can at least earn a living, because here's a guy who comes and says I am broke; I've got a family and you start worrying about the possibility of a suicide, and all that."

Did he or any of his colleagues ever think about the Lieberthal patients who very definitely became suicidal? Many of them had families as well.

"Just one second," I cautioned. "His story about being broke seems quite improbable. The information I got was that in his year working for the Irish Army, which ended, I think, about eight months before he applied to be reinstated, he probably earned close to a million rand."

"Well, we don't have that information. I'm being very open with you. So then I phoned Professor Robert Golele, the head of the Orthopedic Department at the Medical University of South Africa, just outside Pretoria. I said to him, 'Here's a guy who claims to have been rehabilitated. He's remorseful; he's got a family; we are colleagues; we have to try and reinstate him back, but we don't want to let him loose on the public without supervision where he can mess up. So we want to ensure that when he operates, there will be other senior people there to watch him. Let's give the guy a chance'."

The head of that department told him that Lieberthal could not be considered for a post because there had been "so many negative reports" about him. Mariba asked Professor Golele if there was any other head of orthopedics in the country who would be prepared to take Lieberthal for a year or two, depending on the reports. He never got any feedback. So he phoned the Council's administration to say, "My attempts to reinstate this person are failing because nobody will touch him with a barge pole."

As head of the Board that directly controlled doctors, was it right for Mariba to be acting as Lieberthal's unofficial employment agent?

"So, as the situation is now, I don't know where Dr. Lieberthal is; whether he's employed; whether he's sitting at home or what he's doing. I have no clue." Nonsensically, he added, "You might know."

It was incredible that the Council didn't know where he was. Shouldn't it have kept an eye on him to ensure that he didn't get up to anything like the Irish Army caper again? It once "lost" a file involving 32 complaints against him. Had it now lost the doctor himself?

Four months later, when I asked Advocate Mkhize if he knew where Lieberthal was, he replied, "It's been a while, but I know there were challenges to him getting a placement in the public service, because people heard these things, you know. They worried about him. At some point, he called me and said he's having difficulty getting a placement. Would we consider relaxing the requirements? So I said, 'There's no way we are going to relax them. You must stick to the conditions. It's not our duty to find a job for you. You must find a job for yourself and if you do, you must ensure that your supervisor gets in touch with us'. And we haven't been contacted by anybody who is his supervisor. Our assumption is that he has not been able to find a placement in the public service."

"Does it mean that if he can't find a job in the public service, then he can't work as a surgeon?" I asked.

"Oh yes, that's effectively what it means."

He assured me that the Council's membership of the International Association of Medical Regulatory Authorities would prevent Lieberthal from going to somewhere like Australia and starting up there as an orthopedic surgeon "They would demand that he provides them with a certificate of reference from us," he said. "Without that certificate, they can't register him. If they were to ask for that, then we would tell them the truth, that there are these issues. And if they decided to register him, having been given the facts, then it's their issue."

There would have been few people concerned for Lieberthal if he had never been able to work as a surgeon again. It looked as though the media, rather than the Health Professions Council, had at last brought this about.

Here's hoping that in the future there will be a lot more than three, somewhat reluctant, doctors, who will come forward of their own volition with complaints to the Medical Council when other Lieberthal's are seen to be ruining people's lives. If the Hippocratic Oath is to be worth anything at all, it should include something like: I accept that I have a duty to report any member of my profession to my medical council if I have reason to believe that what they are doing is detrimental to the health of patients and is likely to bring the profession into disrepute. Then the powers that be must not just pay lip service to the Oath, but make it really meaningful by taking prompt action against those who fail to uphold it in its entirety.

In addition, doctors should not be allowed a soft landing because they have been given one of the Health Professions Council's often pathetically lenient sentences. In the more serious cases, they should always go on to face a criminal trial like any other citizen who has committed a comparable offence. Either that, or the weak-kneed HPCSA should lose its jurisdiction over disciplinary action for the medical profession and the normal courts should take over completely.

When you have doctors being judged by their colleagues, justice inevitably suffers.

In his 52 years, Lieberthal chanced his arm on numerous occasions, not only in the medical sphere, but in the criminal world, as well. As a doctor, surrounded by the status associated with the Hippocratic Oath, he was able, figuratively speaking, to "get away with murder."

"I have an ominous feeling that the story of Wynne Lieberthal is not yet over," Katy Katopodis of 702 said, when she heard Lieberthal had been reinstated. "Watch this space," she added.

What happened to the disappearing surgeon? Johannes Nkambule, the Manager of the Medical and Dental Professions Board, told me that Lieberthal, who had been restricted to working in Gauteng Provincial hospitals, appeared before the Executive Committee in April 2007 to complain that he had contacted Professor Lukhele at Wits to arrange for his supervision, without success.

"In general, the negative publicity that followed the removal of his name from the register resulted in practitioners and public institutions not having an interest in being associated with Dr. Lieberthal," he said. "Lieberthal expressed concern that there was no collaboration between the Board and public hospitals to ensure that he could comply with the conditions of his re-instatement. To help him, the Committee altered his restrictions so that he could practice in any position at any public hospital."

It was only early in 2008 that the Council appears to have discovered that Lieberthal had been working at the 300-bed St Elizabeth Hospital in Lusikisiki since June 2007. Ignoring the Council's requirement that he should be supervised by a senior surgeon, he set up his own orthopedic unit there because the hospital didn't have one. The hospital, which is in one of the poorest parts of the country near Port St Johns, comes under the Eastern Cape Provincial Health Department. And, because it was in such an out of the way spot, the chances were that nobody there had heard about Lieberthal's pot-holed track record.

When I questioned Mariba about this appointment, he replied, "He got very good commendations from his colleagues who worked with him, some professor who was a surgeon there. All went well, which is something positive." He spoke of this as if it was an achievement the Medical Council could be proud of.

I asked him how Lieberthal could possibly have been properly supervised if he had set up his own orthopedic department, and Mariba said he did not have the "details" of what had happened at Lusikisiki. That was how well they were monitoring the elusive medic.

"Presumably you wanted him supervised by an orthopedic surgeon?" I persisted.

"That would have been the preferred status, but the problem was, he couldn't get a post."

Working in a public hospital, the Professor said, was a form of "community service" for Lieberthal. It's strange logic to punish discredited doctors by putting them in state hospitals. Was it because the less sophisticated people, who would be the ones most likely to attend these institutions, would be unlikely to complain if something went wrong? The poor were effectively being used as guinea pigs for the dregs of the private medical profession to practice on.

In a hushed tone, he added, "Between you and I, I think he will be in the public service for quite some time. The allegations were serious and, at the same time, we wanted to give him a chance to educate his kids; to look after his family and all those things."

A favorable report on Lieberthal's performance was received by the Medical Council from Dr. "Mag" Mohammed Molla. A general practitioner, he was the "accounting officer" and Chief Executive of the St Elizabeth Hospital, so how was he qualified to give the Council the rundown on the operating progress of an orthopedic surgeon? On the basis of his recommendations, the Council decided to relax Lieberthal's restrictions still further.

Once again, the Council's incredibly tolerant approach in dealing with this recalcitrant doctor came into focus. All Lieberthal's long suffering ex-patients and their relatives were given a slap in the face by the HPC's decisions that followed. He was allowed to ignore just about all the restrictions that had been placed upon him for no other reason than his bad reputation made it impossible for him to comply with them.

In February 2008, Lieberthal's restriction, that he had to work under supervision in the public service, was removed even though it appeared that this had never happened. The new registration he was given was "Public Service—specialist." His request to be allowed to assist specialists in the private sector was refused.

I then did what the Council should have done: I delved into what had been happening down at Lusikisiki, a very long way from Lieberthal's old haunts in Johannesburg where he was so well known, and controversy raised its ugly head once again.

Molla told me in May 2008 that, although Lieberthal had started an orthopedic unit at his hospital, he had done all his major operations at the Nelson Mandela Academic Hospital in Umtata, about 130 kilometers away, under the supervision of Professor Chris Macconache. If this was the case, then why had Lieberthal not asked the Professor to send regular reports on his progress to the Medical Council, as required by his reinstatement conditions?

The answer became clear when I phoned the Professor's wife Jenny shortly after I had spoken to Molla. She was a sister running a clinic in Umtata. "My husband had been in and out of hospital with leukemia for two years before he died last December," she said. An orthopedic surgeon, he had headed the Bedford Orthopedic Hospital, which was part of the Nelson Mandela Umtata complex.

Asked whether he had ever supervised operations done by Lieberthal, she said, "I think I know who you are talking about, but I don't think my husband was involved with him, in any way. He applied to come and work at Bedford, and I think my husband smelt a bit of a rat. He started checking references and there were some very unfavorable reports."

Three months after I spoke to Molla, Lieberthal had moved to Witbank, a smelly town East of Johannesburg where the air was heavily polluted from dust from the coal mines in the area. Few people would work there by choice. It was much closer than Lusikisiki to Lieberthal's home in Johannesburg, so that was evidently the attraction for the surgeon who was persona non grata at most hospitals. There, he got a job as Head of the Orthopedic Department at the Witbank Provincial Hospital.

In the past, patients arriving at Lieberthal's opulent rooms, opposite the Rosebank Clinic, had been impressed by the sign writing on the glass entrance door. "Dr. Wynne Lieberthal. INC. MB MCh. Dip. A. Med. FCS (SA) Orth. ORTHOPEDIC SURGEON Specializing in Spinal Disorders," Now people were wondering how long it would be before Lieberthal would be allowed to return to private practice, and those impressive qualifications would once again be luring unsuspecting patients into his web of life-threatening deceit.

Chapter 24

A Doctor In More Ways Than One

In the murky background, hidden behind all the other more sensational things that had been going on in Lieberthal's life, another of his skeletons was being rattled, but not very effectively, it would seem. The police were taking so long that it looked as though this investigation would fizzle out in much the same way as the one several years earlier, when the life insurance companies tried to convict him over the dread disease swindle. Was this surgeon going to set a new standard for that cat with nine lives? In medical circles, he had already given the word "doctor" its other obnoxious meaning.

The criminal justice system was turning out to be even more doctor-friendly to our resourceful specialist than the Medical Council had been. How could the police possibly expect any prosecution to stick in court if they took more than six years to complete what appeared to be a clear cut case, where the records should have been easily available? Witnesses can forget what happened; leave the country; or even die when things are drawn out to this extent. Not that six years was a definite cutoff time, because, when I last inquired, the investigation was still going on. Mr. Plod would certainly have been the right name for the lead detective.

The Star broke the story in April 2003 under the eye-catching headline: "Surgeon robbed us, says hospital." It began: "He says he undertook operations in state hospitals for free, out of the goodness of his heart." Yet, Dr. Wynne Lieberthal was being investigated for charging nearly double the standard price for the surgical prostheses he used in operations."

The newspaper described how Lieberthal had set up a close corporation, Ensemble Trading, which, according to the Johannesburg Hospital records, was listed as a supplier of instrumentation used in most of his operations. In one operation alone that he did at the hospital in February 2002, he made a profit of R55 000 on the hardware used.

Ensemble's banking details listed the number of Lieberthal's practice in Rosebank as the contact number for the person who opened the account and the address of his practice was the same one given for Ensemble. At the Companies and Intellectual Property Registration Office in Pretoria, the paper found that Lieberthal was listed as having 100% of the shares.

Ensemble bought the instrumentation from Stryker Osteonics, where the address given was also that of Lieberthal's Rosebank practice. According to The Star, there were 22 cases of overcharging by Lieberthal being investigated by auditors at the Gauteng Shared Service Centre and by the police at the Commercial Crimes Unit. Accounts already scrutinized showed that the Johannesburg Hospital was overcharged by Ensemble to the tune of R250 000 in just five operations. In one case, the hospital was charged R93 000 for hardware, when the Stryker Osteonics" price to Ensemble was only R55 000.

Lieberthal's attorney told the paper that Lieberthal had sold his interest in Ensemble in November 2000. This was refuted by an affidavit from a Stryker representative, who stated the doctor had been responsible for settling its invoices to Ensemble as recently as February 2002.

Sagie Pillay, the chief executive of the Hospital, was quoted in The Star as saying that the overcharging and conflict of interest were discovered the previous year, when it was noticed that certain bills for prostheses in orthopedics were excessively priced.

"We were cheated and we want our money back," he told the paper.

Pillay told me that it was while reviewing hospital expenditure that they discovered what Lieberthal had been up to. "When I confronted him, he denied that he owned Ensemble or had anything to do with it. In a hospital, doctors are gods and nobody tends to question their judgment if they ask for a particular prosthesis."

There were "numerous doctors and other members of staff", who said he was doing the wrong thing, asking Lieberthal to leave the hospital because he was "such a brilliant surgeon." Since then, Pillay had been approached to let him return. "Some people say we provide a rubbish service at this hospital and it's my job to change that perception. So you can imagine what people would say if I allowed him back after all the problems he caused. He cost this hospital R6-million in the Du Plessis case, which could have been better spent on patient care."

A Gauteng Health Department official told me that if you work in a state hospital, it is illegal for you to buy goods or services for the hospital from your own company. Her department had given all the Lieberthal documents to the police. From then on, the case bounced around as if nobody wanted to touch it. It began life at the Hillbrow Police station, which was in the same area as the hospital, under Docket No 223/03/2003. Then it was passed to the Specialised Commercial Crime Unit in central Johannesburg. In this unit, the detectives worked closely with the prosecutor assigned to the case to hopefully bring the matter to a successful conclusion in court.

The investigating officer was Captain Zanzele Sithole so, in April 2008, I asked him what was happening about the case. He said it concerned an amount of R24-million. I found it difficult to believe that the profit on prostheses could have reached such a vast sum, so I asked for more details. The detective suddenly went into reverse gear like somebody who begins telling a crude joke in mixed company and then realizes he might offend. "I'm not at liberty to divulge that. It would be as good as telling you the contents and the merits of my investigation. Watch this space."

His boss, Superintendent Rose Schickerling, the Serious High Profile Group Head, said, "The docket is still under investigation, that's as much as I can tell you." Almost a year later, she referred me to Advocate Leanna Fick, an exceptionally obliging public servant, especially for someone who worked with the police.

"Sir, the matter used to be one of my cases. *Sjoe!* I think it was already in 2004, 2005," she said. "I don't know why the police referred you to me. I received a statement from the then investigator, Captain du Toit that indicated that the original documents and docket were lost. At that stage, I then closed the case that was on my name."

I gave her the Hillbrow docket number that I had and she said she thought this had been her case. "From what I can remember, it involved hip replacements for which he had billed the Johannesburg Hospital after getting them a lot cheaper. I understand there was a second case that is still running, but I'm not the prosecutor in that matter."

She told me the new prosecutor was Advocate Alma Potgieter and added, "As far as I understand, they are still struggling to finalize the investigation, because portions of the documents got lost at the forensic investigators, and they had to reconstruct them. I'm not too sure what was reconstructed. I think it would be better if you speak to her."

The investigations, one or more of them had now been ineffectively stumbling along for ages. This was not unusual in her Unit, Superintendent Schickerling told me, for cases to take this long, as there were several other ones that had been on the go since 2003. If that was the norm, it was a sad reflection on this specialized unit that was supposed to be there to clean up business.

"I'm still waiting for the investigating officer to come back to me in respect of certain instructions I gave him," Schickerling added.

The Lieberthal case was a touchy subject for Captain Sithole, judging by his reaction when I phoned him after speaking to Potgieter. Incensed, he said, "You keep phoning me. I said I will get back to you as soon as I hear something."

"I phoned you about a year ago, I think," I reminded him.

"Remember, the decision to prosecute doesn't lie with me, it lies with the public prosecutors."

It was always somebody else who had to make further inquiries or who had to decide whether or not to prosecute, no matter whom I spoke to. Worse still was the very disturbing fact that the original docket and documents had just disappeared.

In 2009, the country's Safety and Security Minister Nathi Mthethwa told South Africa's Parliament that 668 dockets went missing or were stolen in the previous 12 months. That was a 56 percent increase on the previous year. Those were the ones they counted, but the problem was probably much greater than that. You would think a police force would have a system to enable it to hold somebody accountable when this happened? The disappearing dockets disease had become a regular feature of police investigations into the doctor's nefarious activities over the years. No wonder the latest case was going nowhere. Had Lieberthal been aware that this arm of the law was suffering from a serious case of muscular dystrophy, he would have been absolutely delighted.

As far as I know, he was able to laugh this one off, just like he had been able to do with all his other money-making schemes that somehow were never officially branded as crimes. He was never prosecuted for this.

Apparently, it did not concern the provincial hospitals at Lusikisiki and Witbank that Lieberthal was still being investigated by the Police when he was employed there. The Medical Council had also ignored this very serious aspect of Lieberthal's behavior.

In defense of their crooked colleagues, the theme song among many government officials was that "people are innocent until proved guilty in court." Did this justify employing a doctor, of all people, who was already suspected of committing a serious fraud against another provincial hospital? Or was it the policy that one more employee with a suspect background was not going to make any difference?

Chapter 25

HPC's Own Problem Doctor

The Health Professions Council of South Africa's 2006/7 annual report was an impressive-looking document, as well produced as any of those sent out by the country's major companies. It recorded the activities of what was said to be one of the largest health regulatory councils in the world, representing 23 professions with over 125 000 registered members, excluding students.

Lieberthal was not the only doctor who got high on Pethidine. It was the drug of choice for many of them. According to the President Dr. Nicky Padayachee's contribution, "Cases of Pethidine abuse by health professionals continue to be reported and pose a continued challenge to the Health Committee."

This was followed by confusing gobbledygook that was hardly what one would expect in a President's message. "Thirty new cases of impairment were recorded during the year, including 12 for substance abuse. The Committee's participatory approach is bearing fruit as 12 cases of practitioners were revoked and the practitioners were declared fully rehabilitated by the Committee."

Tendai Dhliwayo, the Communications Officer, deciphered this verbiage for me by saying the 12 were part of the 30 and all of them involved Pethidine abuse. The 12 were not struck off the register. "Rather, the Committee adopted a way of keeping these practitioners in the system by establishing help lines so that the practitioners involved are steered away from the habit," he said.

Once again, the Council only appeared to be concerned with the welfare of its addicted members. What about their patients, who would continue to be treated by doctors who could well, be high on Pethidine or some other drug? And what about the doctors who did not bother to use the help line?

It had got so bad that, according to Padayachee, "The Council has recommended to the Registrar of the Medicines Control Council that the use of Pethidine be restricted to hospitals and medical institutions only." How this was going to prevent doctors from getting at the stuff, it was difficult to imagine.

The Council had its own festering sore that was hardly a recommendation for a body that professed to police the medical profession. It was something that would never get into any of the annual reports. It concerned Padayachee himself, so he was in no position to criticize doctors for getting bombed from time to time, whether it was on Pethidine or anything else.

In May 2006, the South African Medical Journal carried an article by Chris Bateman in which Padayachee was accused of being drunk during an overseas trip. The article disclosed that the Health Professions Council had closed ranks around its President over his "wayward behavior."

When asked to comment, Padayachee told the Journal he "did not take alcohol as it interfered with the new psychiatric medicine he was on that could induce symptoms similar to drunkenness."

One eyewitness was quoted as saying, "You could smell the alcohol on his breath. He reeked of it," and he was prepared to back this in an affidavit, if asked.

The report was based on accounts by members of a "relationship building" delegation to Switzerland in June 2005, headed by the South African Minister of Science and Technology Mosibudi Mangena. Padayachee resigned shortly afterwards, as the Medical Research Council's Executive Director of Research, for what he described as "unrelated prior health and workload reasons."

The Medical Council just plastered over this very serious wound to its standing, and set a shocking example as a body that was supposed to uphold the ethics of the medical profession. "They decided that, as he wasn't practicing, he could not be disciplined," Bateman told me. "He never complained to us about the story."

In keeping with the profession's hush-hush approach, the discussions about Padayachee were held in camera and no statement was issued by the Council.

Two years earlier, Padayachee was removed from the HPCSA as one of its nominees by the South African Universities Vice Chancellors Association. This followed his resignation as Dean of the Health Sciences faculty at the University of Cape Town, after "a controversy-laden tenure and a memorable graduation ceremony at which he struggled to read names and remain steady on his feet."

He was appointed to the Medical Council by Health Minister, Dr. Manto Tshabalala-Msimang, who had also been in the newspapers, accused of taking to the bottle. Padayachee began his five-year term as President of the Council in May 2004.

The SA Medical Journal is an independent monthly publication, owned by the South African Medical Association, a sort of trade union for doctors. Its editor, Professor 'JP' van Niekerk, told me, "We had quite a bit of flak before the story was published because people got wind of it. We decided to publish because it concerned somebody in high office and it was true."

The Council's motto on its letterheads is "Protecting the public and guiding the professions," but it would seem that there were far too many people outside the medical profession who believed the reality was that the Council guides the public and protects the professions.

Chapter 26

Psychopath

You would have thought that with his brilliant mind, Lieberthal would have learnt his lesson by now. You would have thought he would have realized that even the Medical Council that had been so willing to forgive his many transgressions, might eventually revoke his right to practice as a doctor completely, unless he changed his ways.

You would have been wrong. His Mr. Hyde side could not stop him from destroying lives all over again. And the Medical Council could not change either. It just let him go on operating, as it had done before, while the complaints were coming in thick and fast.

It looked as though Cotterell, the manager of the Rosebank Clinic, got the diagnosis of Lieberthal spot on when he told me, "I think he's a psychopath."

Canadian criminal psychologist, Professor Robert Hare, created a test to determine whether somebody is a psychopath, and Lieberthal certainly ticked enough boxes to qualify.

The list included characteristics such as glibness and superficial charm; lack of remorse; callousness and lack of empathy; all of which were experienced by most of Lieberthal's patients.

Another one was criminal versatility, which was certainly part of Lieberthal's makeup.

The Telegraph in Britain quoted Hare, who had studied people with psychopathy for decades, as saying, "It stuns me that it is possible to have people who are so emotionally disconnected that they can function as if other people are objects to be manipulated and destroyed, without any concern."

In July 2010, again it took the media to flush out Lieberthal. At that stage, 13 new complaints had clocked up against him at the apathetic Medical Council.

It was only when the investigative TV program Carte Blanche exposed his butchery that had been going on at the Witbank Hospital that he promptly resigned.

This was just four months after his easy-going Medical Council had reinstated him as an independent practitioner. It's logical to assume that he must have been messing up people's backs, even before the Council took this step, when it was clearly only thinking about the doctor's welfare, and not anybody he might operate on.

One of the people on this latest list of shame was Pieter Pretorius. Before Lieberthal cut open his back, he could walk, but afterwards, he could only do this for short distances with the aid of crutches.

It was an echo of all the mutilations Lieberthal had been involved in during his career and showed once again how wrong the Council had been to let him return to surgery at all, when he should have been banned for life.

After the first operation, Lieberthal did another one six weeks later, to remove screws that had come loose. This was followed by a third, in which Lieberthal fused a vertebra to two others he had fused before.

The poor man, who lived in Delmas, was reduced to living on painkillers and spending his days sitting in a reclining chair or in bed. His wife Cecilia had become the breadwinner.

Towards the end of 2010, the Council suspended Lieberthal, pending the results of the 13 complaints. Our feisty surgeon's conditioned reflex reacted in the same way he once told the Medical Council he regretted.

He rushed off to the High Court to oppose his suspension. However, a hearing never materialized because, by 2012, the Council had accommodated him, as usual, by allowing him to continue as a doctor. He was reduced to a GP who was not allowed to operate.

Probably in an effort to disappear into obscurity, he moved to Sabie, a forestry town on the banks of the Sabie River in Mpumalanga, near to the Kruger National Park. He had gone a full circle. He was back running his own GP practice for the third time, some 400 kilometers from his old haunts in Johannesburg.

By far South Africa's worst ever surgeon, who had been protected for more than two decades by a Medical Council that inexplicably had a soft spot for him, he finally found that there was one thing from which even he could not escape.

He died suddenly at Sabie on Sunday 5 June 2016 of a heart attack.

He was 61.

Incredibly, his death was followed by a huge outpouring of praise and sympathy from the people of this little country town (Population 10 000).

They clearly had never seen his Mr. Hyde side. The social media tributes painted him as their perfect Dr. Jekyll, far removed from the Lieberthal who had seriously harmed many of his patients, quite a few of whom died not long after they had been in theatre with him.

He was given much acclaim on the town's Facebook page, where Sabie is described as the "Town of the Year." "Today Sabie mourns the loss of a great man," it began, as though Lieberthal had been some kind of saint. "Not only was he our Doctor, but he was our friend. Dr. Wynne Lieberthal—we will remember him as the Doctor who became everyone's friend. A brilliant mind, who was passionate about helping and saving. He lived to serve. May God bless and comfort his family."

Another tribute came from Jenny Moolman who wrote: "Very sad news. Dr. Lieberthal, you will be missed by many. You were a very gentle, caring man and one of the few doctors in today's day and age who would see and attend to your patients any time of the day, even on Sundays. RIP and condolences to your family."

Cathy Rees added to the accolades with: "Wonderful GP and man. Compassionate and caring. Has left a huge hole in Sabie. Love and support to his family."

If only his compassion had extended to saying he was "Sorry" to Mariskca du Plessis, by now confined to a wheelchair, before he died, it would have meant so much to her.

Few of Lieberthal's patients that he operated on would shed a tear, and those that he butchered would no doubt be relieved that he would never again be able to do the same thing to anybody else.

It was said at his disciplinary hearing that the Medical Council had a duty, not only to deal with complaints, but to do its own investigations. In Lieberthal's case, it shirked this duty in many respects, and much of what it did was forced on it by the media publicity. The appalling way it dealt with this doctor while he continued destroying lives on a grand scale, made nonsense of its claim that it is "serious about professional misconduct" and "will stop at nothing to deal with it."

It also rubbished the promise the President Professor Nicky Padayachee made to the Sunday Times in 2004 to do something about what he described as the "inappropriately light sentences" the Council was passing on guilty practitioners. He undertook to ensure there was a "radical overhaul" of Council procedures so that it "could do its job as a watchdog for the public."

BUT NOTHING MUCH CHANGED.

THE END

ABOUT THE AUTHOR

Jon Abbott is a retired, former investigative journalist turned private investigator, based in Cape Town, specializing in business and life insurance. His 600-page report for several life insurance companies formed the basis for this book. He spends a lot of his time as a Consumer Watchdog recording his findings in posts for his hard-hitting, amusing, topical blog the **Dearjon Letter.**

http://dearjon-letter/blogspot.com